Johnson et Al

# MEDI SCHOOL

## AND THE

# RESIDENCY MATCH

**A Post-Match Debrief From Recent Matchers**

2015 Edition

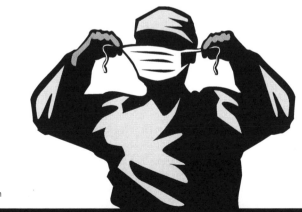

**DoubleU Publishers**
http://www.MedicalMatchBook.com

**Get answers from students who matched at top programs in 2015**

**Contact Info**

| | |
|---|---|
| Web Site | www.MedicalMatchBook.com |
| Facebook | www.facebook.com/medicalmatch |
| Amazon | amzn.com/1514205386 |

*Cover design and typesetting by TopDesign.net*

# CONTRIBUTING AUTHORS

**Harold Callahan**
Detroit, MI
Residency: Dermatology

**Dena Darby**
Colchester, VT
Residency: Family Medicine

**Hank Ng**
Essex Junction, VT
Residency: Internal Medicine

**Burt Johnson**
Pawnee, IN
Residency: Urology

**Samuel Austin**
Springfield, MA
Residency: Anesthesiology

**G. Michael Krauthamer**
USA
Residency: Emergency Med.

**Mairin Jerome**
New York, NY
Residency: Physical Med. & Rehab.

**Alyssa Mendelson**
So. Burlington ,VT
Residency: General Surgery

**Cameron Smith**
Los Angeles, CA
Residency: Internal Medicine

**Tyler van Backer**
Wilmington, VT
Residency: General Surgery

**Whitney Alduron**
Suburban Connecticut
Residency: Anesthesia

**Calvin Barber**
Cardiff-on-the-Sea, CA
Residency: Anesthesia

**Jennifer Tango**
Lancaster, CA
Residency: Emergency Med.

# CONTENTS

Introduction And Purpose      9

Contributing Authors      11

The Classroom Years      16
*Grades, Pre-Clinical Effort, and General Philosophy*

The Boards      24
*USMLE Step 1: Its Value, Importance, and A Little Strategy*

Vacations And Time Off      35
*Summer Between 1st and 2nd Year, Personal Time*

Clerkship Year      40

The Outside World      47
*Extracurriculars, Service, and Research*

4th Year And Away Rotations      55
*Impression and General Experiences*

ERAS Application System      65
*The Personal Statement, Deadlines, and Letters of Recommendation*

The Interview Trail      77
*Program Selection, Logistics, and Pre/Post-Interview Socials*

Interview Day      101
*The Ultimate Purpose, Asking Questions, Being Caught Off Guard, Post-Interview Communication*

Potpourri & Story Time      133

Index      143

# DISCLAIMER

This book is designed to provide information to our readers. It is provided with the understanding that the publisher is not engaged to render any type of legal or any other kind of professional advice. The content is the sole expression and opinion of the authors, and not necessarily that of the publisher. No warranties or guarantees are expressed or implied by the publisher's choice to include any of the content in this volume. Neither the publisher nor the individual author(s) shall be liable for any physical, psychological, emotional, financial, or commercial damages, including, but not limited to, special, incidental, consequential or other damages. Our views and rights are the same: You are responsible for your own choices, actions, and results. Please consult with a legal professional for consul.

The opinions expressed are those of the authors only and not of the institutions they associate with or have associated with in the past or will associate with in the future. None of the content is to be construed as or implied to be professional advising.

This book is intended to provide general information on a particular subject and is not an exhaustive treatment of such subjects. The author and publisher make no express or implied representations or warranties regarding the information herein. Without limiting the foregoing, the author and publisher does not warrant that the content will be error-free or will meet any particular criteria. The publisher and author will not be liable for any special, indirect, incidental, consequential, or punitive damages or any other damages whatsoever, whether in an action of contract, statute, tort (including negligence) or otherwise, relating to the use of information herein.

While every precaution has been taken in the preparation of this book, the publisher and author assume no responsibility for errors or omissions, or for injuries, losses, untoward results, or any other damages that may result from the use of information in this book.

# ACKNOWLEDGMENTS

I'd like to thank all the people that were able to make this book possible. Medical school and the residency application process can feel like a black hole to most applicants, and once you come out the other side, you feel like you have something to share with the future.

I think I was fortunate to have many friends who valued and vehemently protected their personal time. Thus, they were willing to think creatively about how to approach this process most efficiently. Our goal was to share as much information as possible in hopes that future medical students can do the same.

# 1

# INTRODUCTION AND PURPOSE

For better or worse, medical students are very good at jumping through hoops. They are good at following protocols, checking boxes, and taking instruction. They are obedient, hard-working, and generally stay within the lines. It is just this characterization that can make medical school a real grind for many students, when it may not have to be.

I am a mediocre student. I went to my state school for undergrad. I would bet I was in the bottom half of my medical school (by their metrics), also a state school – nothing flashy here. I was willing to admit this the first day of medical school, and will continue to admit it to this day. There are so many more students that are more intelligent and good at putting their heads down and grinding out 12 hours of studying a day.

I knew I wasn't good at that, nor was I interested in ever doing that. Personally, I have a true thirst for knowledge, and that was a big reason why I even showed up to medical school, but I also have an interest in doing things efficiently. With a little planning and focused, strategic efforts, the country bumpkin from rural America was able to have his pick of some of the finest residency programs in the country. And consequently, many of the authors of this book had similar experiences.

The purpose of this book is to help you get some sense of what lies ahead, whether you're about to start your first year of medical school or about to go on residency interviews. Knowing what to expect gives you a sense of expectations and even a chance to plan.

This book makes no attempt to tell you what to do, just merely to provide you with personal experiences from students who have succeeded in the process. In no way should this replace any other form of advising you may get, especially from academic advisers and mentors. This is supplementation, and supplementation from a different angle.

The authors of this book literally just matched, and every topic was relatively fresh in their minds. Their unique perspectives come from someone who has just achieved their goal and can look back on their whole medical school experience in a unique way.

Read it how you want. It's a flexible read - here are some suggestions:

- Read it in order
- Skip from topic to topic
- Follow the entries of one specific author throughout
- Use it as a reference and follow along as you go through school
- Read the funny stories
- Makes good kindling

The book isn't perfect and because it was done on a budget, I fully expect there to be errors. If you do spot some, have any other comments, questions, etc. don't hesitate to get in touch via our contact page at **www.MedicalMatchBook.com**

Best of luck to all!

Burt Johnson and Co.

# 2

# CONTRIBUTING AUTHORS

In order to get some semblance of context to each of the author's contributions and what relevance that may have to your experience, we have profiled each contributor, and additionally indexed where their entries can be found throughout the book.

A challenge with writing an honest book about medical schools and residency programs is that medical specialties can be surprisingly small communities. In order for the authors to be able to share particular details, they were afforded the opportunity to change their names, but the rest of their profile is true. Some were willing to disclose more personal information than others.

While there are so many components that go into evaluating candidates for residency positions, certainly too many to include here, we thought that at the very least, board scores should be included as they can be gatekeepers (and many applicants are interested in actual numbers).

## Harold Callahan

| | |
|---|---|
| Specialty | Dermatology |
| Hometown | Detroit |
| USMLE | Step 1: 250+ |
| Interests | Hockey and Fishing |

## Dena Darby

| | |
|---|---|
| Specialty | Family Medicine |
| Hometown | Colchester, VT |
| Board scores | Step 1: 230 <br> Step 2: 234 |
| Interests | Reading and writing, walking and hiking, friends and family |

## Hank Ng

| | |
|---|---|
| Specialty | Internal Medicine |
| Hometown | Essex Junction, VT |
| USMLE | Step 1: 230 <br> Step 2: 240 <br> CS: F |
| Interests | Soccer |
| Bonus | Going into medical school, he had a rough idea of what he wanted to do. He thought he would end up in internal medicine or pediatrics, and perhaps something after that. Indeed, he always carried a soft spot for hematology and oncology. For better or worse, his specialty choice tinted his view of the rest of medical school. He struggled with internal, family, and pediatrics, before settling on internal medicine. |

## Burt Johnson

| | |
|---|---|
| Specialty | Urology |
| Hometown | Pawnee, IN |
| USMLE | Step 1: 249<br>Step 2: Not disclosed to programs (231)<br>CS: P |
| Grades | Honored 0 pre-clinical courses, 2 clerkships |
| Fun fact | Wanted to be an ESPN Sportscaster |

## Samuel Austin

| | |
|---|---|
| Specialty | Anesthesia |
| Hometown | Springfield, Massachusetts |
| USMLE | Step 1: 270+<br>Step 2: 280+<br>CS: P |
| Fun fact | Everything in the universe literally is – or isn't –. Also, I had a career-ending ankle fracture during the first practice of my senior year of high school wrestling. That'll teach me from ever getting sweaty in Spandex again. |

## G. Michael Krauthamer

| | |
|---|---|
| Specialty | Emergency Medicine |
| Hometown | Unknown |
| USMLE | Step 1: 230 |
| Interests | Boats and my child |
| Bonus | I started medical school with the intention of applying to Psychiatry residency, and it wasn't until August of my fourth year that I decided to apply to Emergency Medicine residencies. Academically, my preclinical grades were solidly average (read: I passed but did not honor any pre-clinical coursework). My Step 1 score was 230, which was a couple points above the mean for the year that I took it. In my clerkship year I honored Family Medicine, |

Psychiatry and Internal Medicine, I passed the others. That said, I had very strong clinical evaluations, which were reflected in my deans letter. I also honored my fourth year rotations, including my sub-internships in Emergency medicine.

## Mairin Jerome

| | |
|---|---|
| Specialty | Physical Medicine & Rehabilitation |
| Hometown | New York City, NY |
| USMLE | Step 1: 186 (Fail) → 216 (retake) |
| | Step 2: 244 |
| | CS: P |
| Fun fact | When I was 18, I welded a small portion of the tram tracks in Amsterdam. More recently, I got to kayak within 30 feet of a family of humpback whales in the Sea of Cortez. Baby humpbacks are super cute and awkward when learning how to breach! |

## Alyssa Mendelson

| | |
|---|---|
| Specialty | General Surgery |
| Hometown | South Burlington, VT |
| USMLE | Step 1 & 2: Mid - 240s |
| Interests | I may or may not be a crazy cat lady |

## Cameron Smith

| | |
|---|---|
| Specialty | Internal Medicine |
| Hometown | Los Angeles, CA |
| Board scores | 235 - 245 |
| Fun Fact | Larry David is my spirit animal. |

## Tyler van Backer

| | |
|---|---|
| Specialty | General Surgery |
| Hometown | Wilmington, VT |
| Boards | 230s |
| Interests | If there's a soccer game, I'm there. Did EMS throughout college/med school, did a research study with national funding, from small town VT ... nothing else too interesting about me. |

## Whitney Alduron

| | |
|---|---|
| Specialty | Anesthesia |
| Hometown | Suburban Connecticut |
| USMLE | Step 1: High 220s<br>Step 2: High 240s |
| Interests | Skiing, road biking, running |

## Calvin Barber

| | |
|---|---|
| Specialty | Anesthesia |
| Hometown | Cardiff, CA |
| USMLE | Step 1: 236 |
| Interests | Rocking out |

## Jennifer Tango

| | |
|---|---|
| Hometown | Lancaster, CA |
| Specialty | Emergency Medicine |
| Step scores | Step 1 – mildly bombed ... damn man problems<br>Step 2 – 249 |
| Interests | Snowboarding is fun until you fall at Lake Tahoe and probably tear your meniscus months before beginning residency...MRI is next week! Wish me luck! ;) Oh yeah, and don't take life too seriously. No one gets out alive! |

# 3

# THE CLASSROOM YEARS

*Grades, Pre-Clinical Effort, and General Philosophy*

## Alyssa Mendelson, General Surgery

You have to think about what you want AFTER medical school and then tailor your classroom years accordingly. If you want to go into something highly competitive like dermatology, radiology, or orthopedic surgery, of course you should try to honor as many classes as possible without wanting to kill yourself in the process. If you want to go into something less competitive, I'm not sure how much they really matter. I personally didn't know what I wanted to go into, so I tried to honor as many as I could just in case I chose a very competitive specialty. All that being said, I know people who honored none of our classes, did well during their clinical years and are applying to competitive specialties. If you want to make it work, you will. You might just have to fight a little harder later on.

## Calvin Barber, Anesthesiology

Did I know what I wanted to do during first year...

Absolutely I knew I wanted to do – Pediatrics, that's what brought me back to medical school. That's what I thought I would do, and a key thing I think for medical school as a whole, is to be really open to everything that comes up. Show up for everything. Try and get engaged with everything. Because sometimes, things surprise you.

I did psychiatry my first 3rd year rotation and loved it. And throughout the whole rest of third year, that was very much the most likely specialty for me. Later on, I did my pediatrics rotation and really didn't enjoy it. I love the patient population, but didn't especially like the pediatricians. I found a lot of the basic pediatrics very boring. Well-child visits... I mean really, it makes no sense that people with at least 8 years of medical training are doing those. It just is not working at the peak of your capabilities. You could train a teenager to do that as a summer job.

> " ... and a key thing I think for medical school as a whole, is to be really open to everything that comes up. Show up for everything. Try and get engaged with everything. Because sometimes, things surprise you."
>
> -*Calvin Barber*

I didn't actually fail anything, but there were times I was sure as hell had. There were times when I thought, "I can't do this, this has been a terrible mistake, this is too hard, I'm too stupid." I think everyone has those periods, and one piece of advice I have is... keep showing up. Just keep showing up. It's very easy to disengage, when you're feeling down. For me, during those times of struggle, just being present... eventually things got better. And that was tough on occasions.

As I dictate this, I'm driving from Los Angeles to some god-forsaken little town in the Central Valley of California at 5 o'clock in the morning. I'm matching into anesthesia - it's fairly competitive but not top end competitive. In that context, I don't think any of my pre-clinical stuff had the slightest bit of relevance, the caveat being that I did not fail anything. That's probably important to a degree. If you flat out fail a course, that will have to be explained. Fortunately, I was not in that position, but I also didn't honor anything of any significance. I did get honors for the public health project, I've dallied with honors in several other courses but didn't honor anything else. And my scores in class were generally about the median - maybe top half of the class, but I don't think any of that actually gets reported from my institution. The only thing that anyone is actually going to pay attention to is whether you fail stuff.

## Harold Callahan, Dermatology

Do grades matter?

This all depends if your school has an AOA process/chapter and how they calculate which students are eligible (usually top 25% of the class). All schools include clerkship grades into this algorithm so they are important. Clerkship grades (3rd year) are very important for this reason.

People will tell you that first year grades are not important and directors do not look at them. Although this is probably true, many schools (my own) include these grades into the AOA calculation. So, if you don't honor a good number of your first year classes, then you can kiss your chances at AOA goodbye. Take home point: If you have AOA, find out what grades are used to calculate the top 25%.

## Whitney Alduron, Anesthesiology

For me I don't think grades during first and second year mattered much. I only honored one of 12 pre-clinical courses (I think) and it didn't seem to have any adverse effect on my ability to get the residency interviews I wanted (and subsequently the match). I think the most frustrating thing with the grading system, at least at my institution, is that you can end up with a 92.5 or a 75.5 and still receive a score of "pass." There is obviously a significant difference between the two grades which is not necessarily reflected in your application. In order to get a 93 there was significantly more work that needed to be put into studying which I didn't feel was necessarily worth it for me. Not to say I didn't try hard and study a lot, but I would've much rather spent my time running or skiing and come out with an 88 or 90 as opposed to studying all the time and focusing on getting a 93.

## Burt Johnson, Urology

In my mind, the purpose of the classroom years is to build a solid foundation of knowledge. When it comes directly to the residency application process, and the criteria upon which residency directors make their decisions, I think preclinical grades have very little influence and may not even be in the top 10 in terms of importance.

The preclinical years serve to build knowledge in order to optimize your ability to practice medicine and hopefully maximizing your Step 1 board score. Ultimately, it also forms the foundation of both clinical and basic science knowledge that you can translate into the clerkship and fourth year with away rotations and eventually in practice. The more learning you can do during the first two preclinical years, the better off you will be in terms of the amount of refreshing and refurbishing of your knowledge you need to do in the future.

The only instance I believe where preclinical grades factor in at all is in determining your AOA honor society status. My understanding is that in order to be eligible, you need to be at least in the top 25% of your graduating class. Each school calculates or takes into account different things when calculating whether in the top 25%. Typically it's a combination of preclinical grades and clinical clerkship grades. The AOA status is more of a binary object, you either are AOA positive or negative. I wasn't AOA, and I think that may have prevented me from getting some interviews at big-name research programs, for example. For example I didn't get an interview Johns Hopkins or Penn or Cleveland Clinic, I would speculate that lack of AOA was the reason. However I'm just speculating - it could've been a whole host of other factors as well as urology being a very competitive field with a large amount of applicants and few positions.

*"There were times when I thought, "I can't do this, this has been a terrible mistake, this is too hard, I'm too stupid." I think everyone has those periods, and one piece of advice I have is ... keep showing up. Just keep showing up."*

*-Calvin Barber*

My personal approach to the preclinical years was to treat the preclinical years as if it was a regular job. Before going medical school I was gainfully employed as an engineer. I went to work every day and left at 5 o'clock. Maintaining a regimented structure in medical school was important for me to remain disciplined and keep adding knowledge every day.

What I did was I would come to school at 7:15 every day even though lectures would typically start at 8:00, and I would just work until 5 o'clock daily. After 5, I would leave my stuff at school and bring nothing home. After 5, it was time for exercise, fun, family, eating, and just taking care of the rest of my life. This division helped me to stay disciplined while I was at work/school to make sure that I was focused, working, and not being distracted. This disciplined approach made the fire hydrant of knowledge not seem so overwhelming. It was a nice balance of giving my best effort and maintaining my fulfilling, sane life. I wasn't specifically trying to honor every class, simply just trying to learn without regard for scores and competition.

I never honored any preclinical classes, and at first I was a little worried but realized that it didn't matter much toward the ultimate goal which was getting a residency spot in my preferred program in my preferred specialty. Therefore, I prioritized not overextending during this period of medical school, and I think this served me well because I wasn't burned out and I had plenty of energy left for summer activities, clerkship year, and towards USMLE Step 1 studying.

The other item of advice for the preclinical years is to be very aggressive about exploring every specialty you can. The sooner you discover a specialty you love, or one you hate, the better. Make this a priority because the students that were fortunate to have decided relatively early were able to get involved in projects or have experiences that made them significantly more competitive than applicants that were scrambling at the start of 4th year.

## Cameron Smith, Internal Medicine

In hindsight, there are many things that I would have changed about my first 1.5 years in the classroom. First, I would have altered my studying methods. I began medical school, as most perfectionist medical students do, attempting to memorize every detail of every PowerPoint slide or lecture that I was given. Somehow I managed to get through even the toughest courses in college. However, the amount of information in medical school makes this task impossible.

If I could step into a time machine, I would go back and work diligently on identifying the material that seemed higher yield. Easier said than done, it takes experience.

As far as grades go, I think that it's best to give every course 110% and have an organized structure by which you study. However, in hindsight, I did stress too

*"People will tell you that first year grades are not important and directors do not look at them. Although probably true, many schools (my own) include these grades into the AOA calculation."*

*-Harold Callahan*

much over gaining honors in every class. Again, because we are perfectionists and competitive individuals, we naturally expect the best results and often are dissatisfied with anything less than perfection. However, balance is key. Give every course 110% while maintaining a balanced lifestyle. If you enjoy video games, work it in for 30-60 minutes at the end of the night. If you like the gym, don't give it up to gain an extra hour or two of study time. And in the end if you don't get the honors, know that grades are probably not even on the top five list of ways that residency programs will evaluate you.

## Tyler van Backer, General Surgery

Depends what your goals are. If you want to go to a top-tier residency program (e.g. MGH, the Brigham, etc.), then yes, they do. If you would also be okay with matching in another academic or community program, they probably matter less so. Looking at the top-tier and some of the more competitive programs, they consider AOA status, which is based on grades (among other things). I was asked in one residency interview why I had only passed a rotation, instead of honoring it. I also didn't interview at the most competitive schools, so there's probably some selection bias there, as well.

Best use of time: Studying for exams and doing well in school is obviously important, but staying sane is, as well. I had a couple of extra-curricular activities and made sure to try to keep up a good workout routine to help my sanity. I enjoy volunteering, so that was a good outlet, as well. Sometimes, I did feel like I was spread a little thin, though.

## Jennifer Tango, Emergency Medicine

I wouldn't put a lot of stock in pre-clinical grades. Granted, it absolutely depends what specialty you're pursuing. If you want to be an orthopedic surgeon or a dermatologist, it would be in your best interest to honor some classes! But if you want to be a pediatrician or family doctor, it's more important to learn the vitals of how to be a good clinician.

The only thing I honored in the first 3 years of medical school was a public health project (was that because other people were working on it too??? Who knows!). Eventually I became a 4th year and stopped caring what other people wanted me to say or to think or to learn. I have honored every rotation but two in my fourth year. Was I all of a sudden a much better student than during third year? I doubt it. I think I just started learning what I was interested in, didn't already know, or knew was a deficiency in my learning. Be a dedicated learner and close the gaps in your knowledge. You'll do alright.

## Mairin Jerome, PM & R

Initially, I was very worried about honoring preclinical courses. A student in the class above me told me the grades don't matter and that 3rd year clerkships are more important. This was true and took a lot of pressure off, with the caveat that a correlation exists between course performance and Step 1 board scores. Be mindful of mastering content for Step 1.

For the residency match process, pre-clinical grades don't matter all that much for most students. No one ever asked me about them, and as far as I know, they are not used for screening, save for being an AOA member. Grades can be useful personally for understanding how you are grasping the material overall, which could potentially be extrapolated to determine your preparedness for Step 1.

In hindsight, I wish I had spent less time pursing interesting extracurricular activities (interest groups, volunteering, Schweitzer fellowship), and more time on Step 1 Board preparation. The activities were all fun and interesting, and frankly what led me to medical school, but I was a non-traditional student with a background that was weaker in the sciences. If you are in a similar situation starting out, you may be better served to spend more time studying and less time doing things that were interesting, fun, and probably more meaningful. In my view, the first 2 years of medical school are there to prepare you for Step 1, a critically important test.

## Hank Ng, Internal Medicine

The first 1-2 years in the classroom seemed monumental at the time, but in hindsight they didn't carry much significance. I didn't honor a single class, but passed all of them comfortably. I was never asked about any of my classes on interviews. My feeling is that classes only help in the sense of honoring and then having that contribute towards AOA. Unfortunately I have nothing to offer on that front, but keep reading, I am sure some AOA people will share their experiences.

I tried my best in the classes, just wasn't able to honor any of them. I felt that I built a solid base of knowledge from the classroom – the first piece towards studying for Step 1. And there was definitely some pimping on clinical rotations that made me reach back to the classroom. I would say the biggest secondary benefit besides the knowledge in the classroom was getting to know the actual clinicians that taught some of our classes. Seeing some of these individuals in the lecture hall and lab, we were slightly more at ease when they started to pimp us in the patient halls on rounds. In other cases, it was an opportunity to find someone of interest to shadow, pursue research, or some other extracurricular activity.

I don't know how your medical school worked, but for the most part we had exams on Mondays. It was the catch 22 of having more time to study, but no weekends. Rather, we crammed our weekends into Monday afternoon/evening. Tradition dictated a trip to the Irish pub Ri Ra's, and whenever we finished a class – broffet (just a good group of guys stuffing their faces at an all you can eat Chinese buffet with a guarantee of regret and quality time on the john).

## Samuel Austin, Anesthesia

In my experience, preclinical grades only matter so much as to prepare you for Step 1, which therefore builds an important foundation for clinical medicine. Take your classes seriously as it is simultaneously the best way to "study" for the boards and allow you to learn how to take the best care of patients. If you find going to lecture works well, then do that. If you don't get much out of lecture, don't go. You pay a lot of money to attend medical school so make the best use of your time.

# 4

# THE BOARDS

*USMLE Step 1: Its Value, Importance, and A Little Strategy*

## Alyssa Mendelson, General Surgery

Board scores are important, but not the end all be all. They can be used to determine AOA status, some programs during the application season will "filter" their lists and only interview board scores above a certain number. Those are really only for the most competitive programs. If you want to just end up in NYC and don't care if you go to Columbia or a less "prestigious" program, just get your score to the national average. If you can't do that, work your ass off in clerkships and round out your application in other ways.

At this point, you all know how to study. You can't really get into medical school not knowing how to study. Everyone will tell you certain programs or textbooks are the "best," but we all have different learning styles, so just know how you learn. If you like videos, do DIT and pathoma. If you are a reader/notetaker, just hammer First Aid and supplement with other resources you like. If you have no idea how you learn best, I'd recommend getting in touch with your medical student education office and have them help you develop a schedule and find appropriate resources.

Often times, your school will offer tutoring. You need to make a schedule and stick to it. You can't futz around. It's too much information and you need to cover all of it, likely more than once. Take practice tests, do as many questions as you can. Lastly, once or twice a week, DO SOMETHING FUN.

> *"I had a whole week where I ate cheesy rice, frosting out of the container, and had somewhere in the neighborhood of 5 cups of coffee per day. Don't do that."*
>
> *-Alyssa Mendelson*

The process will suck the life out of you, so fight back and try to maintain having an actual human being's life. Also, try to exercise, eat healthy, and get enough sleep. I had a whole week where I ate cheesy rice, frosting out of the container and had somewhere in the neighborhood of 5 cups of coffee per day. Don't do that. I felt like shit and had an awful study week. Go to the grocery store, I promise it's worth losing a little bit of study time. (Step 1 = mid 240s)

I took Step 1 about two weeks before clerkships started. Having that free time was a priority for me. I knew I would need to recover. A couple of classmates and I went to Florida and hung out at Harry Potter world drinking Butterbeer for a week. It was perfect.

## Samuel Austin, Anesthesia

Unfortunately board scores seemed to be an important piece of the puzzle for interview selection. I hate the idea of standardized tests, as they only quantify – and poorly in my opinion – one aspect of intelligence, whereas there are many forms of intelligence (e.g., social, emotional, etc…) that are essential to be an excellent doctor.

Realize the exam is to assure basic competence for medical practice by passing the test; it seems that the numerical score achieved after 196 doesn't reveal much more than an individual's aptitude for taking a multiple choice test. With that said, my best advice is to play the game and score the highest that you can on these exams despite their failure to demonstrate many of your great personal characteristics. You're a professional hoop-jumper by this point and you can jump through this one, too. I was fortunate to earn high marks, and it definitely opened doors for me despite my sentiments about their utility. (Step 1 = 270+)

## Burt Johnson, Urology

This is an absolutely vital exam. I don't intend to belabor an already obvious point, but I cannot emphasize how important it is to dedicate yourself to Step 1. You don't want to get your score back and think there was something more that you could've done. Right now you may want to apply into a less competitive specialty, but many before you have changed their minds. Despite initially wanting to do a less competitive specialty, I lived in fear of falling in love with a specialty that required high board scores. I just sucked it up and studied properly.

While it doesn't necessarily estimate your quality as a doctor, the reality is that it's a door-opener and a door-closer. It is of utmost priority to make sure that as many doors are open to you as possible, especially given the relative increase in number of medical graduates and residency applicants, US MDs, DOs, and IMGs.

Let's say you totally ace Step 1 and you decide to do family medicine or pediatrics, historically specialties that place less emphasis on Step 1 scores, what's the harm? None, you've basically just solidified some medical knowledge that you will use somewhere down the road. The beauty of doing your best on Step 1 - you're not pigeonholed into a specialty you don't want. This is not to say you need to get an amazing score on Step 1, you need to just do your best.

Just as pre-clinical coursework, I treated preparation just like a job: 7:30 AM to 5 PM every day just hammering away, sometimes on my own, sometimes with my study group. Group studying is valuable in that it holds you accountable to show up somewhere and get through the material even when you don't feel like it.

Importantly, you need to take care of your body and brain, you need to fuel like a professional. Professional athletes go on the field and all you see is their gameday performance. However, they practice every day, lift weights, and do all sorts of drills to prepare themselves. Their preparation also extends off the field to game film and taking complete care of their bodies with regards to what they eat how they sleep. Be a professional about Step 1, take care of your body, and exercise - the fundamentals for optimizing your brain performance. (Step 1 = 249)

## Harold Callahan, Dermatology

Keep it [studying] simple and be fast. First aid and UWorld are all you need. Memorize the book. Do laps through the book. Do all of the questions multiple times."

## Hank Ng, Internal Medicine

Step 1 is for some reason the biggest one. I don't know why, Step 2 seems much more relevant clinically. My scores were only brought up once in the interview process.

There were many approaches to Step 1 in my class. Some started studying a couple months out (4 months or so), skipping one of our last classes and podcasting lectures. Others didn't start studying until our designated study time, which was about 2 months.

I tried a bunch of different products to study for Step 1. In hindsight, I wouldn't have used Doctors In Training, I would have done all of Goljan. I really liked Pathoma and obviously the UWorld question bank and First Aid. I might have done another question bank – maybe Kaplan. My recommendation is to try a bunch of different resources, and stick with whatever works for you.

Some of my friends loved Doctors In Training, I didn't like it, but I already invested so much time and the peer pressure element of it, I completed the course anyways. I learn best by doing questions and getting them wrong, so I would have done more question banks.

Balance is necessary during the study period. I probably started studying 3 months before my exam date, and then really hit the books 1.5 months out. It was really important that I go to the gym every day, to take breaks to watch a show or eat lunch, there was no way to study 10 hours straight. (Step 1 = 230)

## Whitney Alduron, Anesthesia

Board scores are important simply because it allows you to be compared to other medical students across the country. That being said, for anesthesia it is only important to do around the national average or better. I did average on Step 1 (high 220s) and above average on Step 2 (high 240s). Improvement looks good on an application.

When I took Step 1, I was debating between internal medicine and anesthesia. I took a look at the board score ranges and saw that both were around the national average so I didn't necessarily feel that I needed to do exceptionally well in order to match at a good program. I moved my Step 1 test forward by three days and took two full weeks off and went on to back to back ski trips in Montana and California before starting clerkship.

This was the best thing I could have done for myself, and I'm very glad I had a full two week vacation before starting clerkships.

## Tyler van Backer, General Surgery

Board scores are very important. Programs say they look at the entire application, but it's not possible to look at every single application, so there are cut-offs. I was told that sometimes it's the secretary who looks at Step 1 and if the score is below a defined cut-off, the application is discarded.

If you do average or above on Step 1, it will get your foot in the door, but it's also up to the rest of your application to get you an interview. It depends on the program for Step 2. Some require it and others don't care as long as you pass. If you submit your Step 2 score, make sure it is better than Step 1. The national average changes each year, but 230 is a good goal to be above. Of course, there are people who match with a lesser score, and to be at a top-tier program you'll need a higher score.

I knew I wanted to do surgery before medical school. Obviously, try to do your best, but if you know you want to do a competitive specialty (orthopedics, dermatology, integrated programs, etc.), it becomes that much more important to really ace your boards.

Timing-wise, I started reading through the books I used to correlate with class material (First Aid) about 4 months before my exam date. I began dedicated studying for Step 1 about 3 months before my test date.

During the studying months, set up fun things to do to look forward to. I would break the day into two sections and go to the gym between. One day a week, I tried to not pick up a book/look at my computer (easier said than done) and found that it helped me stay fresh for the 6 other long days each week. The day before the exam, also try to not study at all, or at least limit yourself to just studying during the morning. (Step 1 = 230s.)

## Mairin Jerome, PM & R

HUGELY important. How you perform on Step 1 will greatly impact whether or not your application is even considered at a residency program.

I failed Step 1. It was awful. In retrospect I would have done things much differently. First of all, I would have studied more during the first two years. At my school, and likely others, there is a correlation between pre-clinical coursework and board scores. I passed all of my courses (Pass/Fail curriculum) in the first 2 years, but in the majority of courses, I scored in the bottom 50%.

Top reasons why I failed:

1. Nervous
2. No organized study plan
3. I did the Uworld Question bank, but did not finish it
4. I started an online course, but realized it would take me much longer than recommended, so I abandoned it and just went through First Aid
5. Took 5 weeks to study

I ended up scoring 2 points below failing. This was devastating. I felt like my whole career would be ruined, I was in the bottom 6%of medical students, I must be the worst person ever, etc. Luckily, my dean of students was amazing and talked me out of my panic and connected me with some other students who had failed Step 1, but matched into great specialties. So, it happens. If you fail, don't fret. Your life is not over.

I ended up taking my next clerkship off to study again. I made a more detailed study plan and did a question bank 1.5 times. This time I scored a 216, near the national average.

## Cameron Smith, Internal Medicine

Step 1 scores are crucial. I look at your Step 1 score as a window that will either close or open with regards to future residency options. In general, a score in the 230s will put your foot in the door for the competitive residency programs, while 240 and above will make you more competitive. Above a 250, I don't think scores matter much, your board score is an asset.

That being said, it's important to know that a Step 1 score that falls below the average score of those who have matched into a particular specialty should NOT deter you from applying to that field. There are many people with scores in the 220s who have matched into some of the most competitive specialties. However, if your score is lower, you need to find other ways of standing out.

In my opinion, the most important aspect of studying for Step 1 and Step 2 is doing as many test prep questions as possible. It's obviously important to have the foundation necessary to answer these questions, but I would stress dedicating more time to actually taking timed question blocks over spending exorbitant amounts of time reading information and facts. Practice, not reading, makes perfect.

There were times during medical school when I had family issues going on back home. At the time, it was extremely stressful to balance both med school and family life. I would urge anyone going through any family issues to take a step back from school and manage your personal life if need be.

## Calvin Barber, Anesthesia

In terms of board scores, I think Step 1 is tremendously important. One program where I did in an away rotation, I had a conversation with the chief of anesthesia. He told me that they have a cut off of 230 for Step 1 scores. I think all programs that I interviewed at have a cut off, not all acknowledged that fact. My impression is that there are roughly three levels.

A lot of programs have a cutoff around 220, maybe even lower possibly 210s. The majority of programs have a fairly low average cutoff, but there's probably a handful of programs maybe like UCSF or OHSU, places like Stanford maybe UCLA, that may even use 240 as a cutoff, but that's just my speculation. The key thing is if you're below the cutoff, they simply don't look at your application. A caveat to that is that I interviewed at one place where I think I didn't meet criteria, and my program director at my medical school made a personal phone call and said you should take a look at the whole application here. As a result I did get an interview, and I went there and I did not in any way feel that I was not a strong, competitive candidate. Personal phone calls can potentially get you over that hurdle of a Step 1 cutoff. The issue with that is they have to have an available interview slot.

So Step 1 score, really important. Can you dig yourself out if you score well on Step 2? Yes potentially. Same thing applies - someone will probably have to make a personal call or you will have to make a big effort to get them to look at your application. So is it possible with hard work? Absolutely. Is it potentially crippling for you? Yes absolutely. Just for the record, my Step 1 score is 236 which is not stand out, but it is solid. I think it kept me in the game.

For me, I did Kaplan, the Doctor In Training (DIT) videos, I went through First Aid fairly comprehensively. There are so many stories of how to guarantee success… that you've got to go through First Aid 5 times or you must do this or you've got to do that, they may or may not be true depending on who you talk to and how you learn.

Looking back, the thing that was really useful was doing questions, and I didn't do as many of those as I should have. I got the UWorld Qbank, and I did that with a couple of friends which I think was also key. I didn't do all of the questions, I did about 2000 questions out of some 2500. Honestly, that was where all the high value stuff for me as a learner was and I should have spent more time doing those. The UWorld Qbank I found to be really useful. The explanations, illustrations, images, diagrams were far superior to the other products I tried.

# USMLE Step 2

## Calvin Barber, Anesthesia

As for Step 2, I just did the questions and felt like I was just trying to memorize the answers and it's not the same as talking through questions and five potential answers - why some are right and why some could be wrong. That talking process is really useful for me and I would have done more of that if I could go back and do it again.

## Whitney Alduron, Anesthesia

In hindsight, Step 1 and Step 2 are very different and just because you didn't do well on Step 1 doesn't mean you can't do well on Step 2, although doing well on Step 1 carries over a lot of knowledge to Step 2. Step 2 for me was much easier because it was logical and clinically-based as opposed to rote memorization. I studied six days a week for 3 1/2 weeks for Step 2 and I felt like that was adequate time. I did not use any other materials aside from the UWorld questions and just took practice test after test. I took 3 1/2 weeks to study for Step 2 I studied six days a week and took one day completely off each week I felt it was plenty of time.

## Harold Callahan, Dermatology

My school gave me one month to study. I used it, but definitely didn't study as much as Step 1. This is probably why I didn't do as well. Realistically, it doesn't matter as much for applications as Step 1. If you take it after November, your score will not automatically be uploaded to ERAS, and thus not reported to the programs you are applying to. At this point, it becomes a pass/fail test with regards to your residency application. For most specialties no one asks about Step 2. I personally had 10 dermatology interviews with no Step 2 score loaded and no one asked about it during interviews. My advice is to take it late if you have a good Step 1 score. Taking Step 2 can only hurt you at that juncture.

## Hank Ng, Internal Medicine

I repeated the same study pattern as with Step 1, but with a little less time studying and fewer resources. I used UWorld, First Aid, Kaplan's review book, and Step Up to Medicine. I really liked Kaplan's review book for test taking strategies fused with content. And no, Kaplan does not sponsor me.

It was nice knowing I wasn't going into orthopedics or neurosurgery. I felt like I could study and do my best on the exams without the pressure/fear of needing a certain score to be eligible for that specialty. Or you could look it as me not pushing myself to the limit without having the negative incentive (a little bit of fear is probably good). I had a bunch of friends who went into selective specialties and crushed the boards. They can speak more to the pressure and strategies of those specialties. At the point of Step 1, I was thinking medicine and pediatrics, and by Step 2 I was set on internal medicine.

## Burt Johnson, Urology

Step2 - Urology is an early match so I didn't take Step2CK until after all my residency interviews. As far as I know, no Urology programs require a Step2CK score in order to be ranked. I went on 12 interviews, and I was asked about Step 2CK at none of them. You do have to submit a passing score by the time you start their residency. As a baseline, I had a 249 on Step1. I prepared for Step2 using UWorld questions for 1.5 weeks and ended up scoring a 231 in what was essentially a pass fail situation. For your purposes, this can serve as a bit of a benchmark for how much any base knowledge can carry you from Step1.

## Mairin Jerome, PM & R

I ended up doing much better on Step 2 (I scored a 244 vs. 186 and 216). I did questions throughout third year and ended up going through the question bank at least twice. A friend who also struggled with test taking got tutoring through a professional company. It is outrageously expensive, but ultimately ended up making the investment and I am SO happy that I did too. I never would have considered this for Step 1 because it was so expensive, but in retrospect I wish I had. This is much better than just working with a student from your school. These are people are exceptional studiers and test takers, and if it is not your forte, it is worth the investment.

## Cameron Smith, Internal Medicine

I found Step 2 easier to study for than Step 1. As mentioned earlier, I emphasized doing as many questions as possible. I took one month off to study for Step 2 at the beginning of my fourth year. During that month, about two weeks in, my grandfather passed away and obviously I had to take a few days off. Despite that, I still found it doable to study about 8 hours a day and get through all of the information I wanted to get through. It's important to note that for those going into competitive specialties, an excellent Step 2 score can benefit those with a sub-par Step 1 score. For this reason, I would advise taking Step 2 soon after the clerkship year ends if you want to go into a competitive specialty, and your Step 1 is weak.

## Tyler van Backer, General Surgery

My family medicine clerkship was the last one of my third year and I planned to take Step 2 right after my third year, so I just studied for Step 2 to study for family medicine (minus a couple of school-specific requirements). I then took three weeks after my third year before the start of fourth year to study exclusively for Step 2. The studying time I put in was much less than Step 1, however.

# Hank Ng, Internal Medicine

Somehow I managed to fail Step 2 CS. Don't ask me how – I have done really well in all of our school's clinical skills exams. I retook CS and passed, but that definitely came up in my interview process. And I am sad to say, that definitely prevented me from getting a lot of interviews. I initially applied to 33, some were reaches and others location challenged (I applied to 10 California schools and I am from Vermont, let's just say I really wanted to take my talents there), but only got interviews at 6. I talked with our schools medicine program director and a couple advisors, and they said it was specifically my CS (at the time I had retaken CS, but didn't know if I passed). I applied to another 7 schools and got one more interview.

I will be honest I don't know how I failed in the first place – I guess I am in that elite group of US allopathic medical students (AOA? Who needs that when you can fail CS). And then I passed with the retake without doing anything differently. I am confident I would have gotten more interviews if I had passed it, or had gotten the retake score earlier in the process. I didn't know this, but CS has set reporting periods, so if you take the test within a certain time (say May to mid- July) your score will be reported out in a set period (August to the first week in September ). I had no idea, and if I even thought that failing was a possibility, I would have planned differently. I had the perfect storm of terrible luck. I took the exam in early July and it got my score back early August, right in time to get reported when I released my USMLE scores for ERAS. And my rescheduled exam was September 8th, which just missed the next reporting period. One of my friends took her exam September 6th and got her scores back in early October. I got my scores back December 3rd – I just missed the most recent cutoff – and by that time most interview spots are set. I have no idea if I would have gotten more interviews if I had gotten my passing score in early October like my friend; I would like to think that I would have gotten more, but who knows. It is just getting so competitive for everything, if they have any way to differentiate they use it, not that I can blame them.

Obviously the question came up in all of my interviews: variations of "what happened with Step 2 CS?" or "how did you fail?" I knew this was going to come up, but I really had no answer. All I knew was that I failed the ICS section – which combines history taking, physical exam, and note writing. I have never had a problem at our school's clinical exams and I still have no idea what happened the first time. I wasn't sure how to approach this in interviews, I was honest – saying I have no idea what happened, I tried to joke that maybe I was mean to a patient, forgot to write a note, or the alcohol hand sanitizers were a trap and I should have been washing my hands in the sink.

# 5

# VACATIONS AND TIME OFF
*Summer Between 1st and 2nd Year, Personal Time*

## Calvin Barber, Anesthesia

Between 1st and 2nd year I went to Barbados. I did not do anything that was vaguely medically or clinically related. That was a very good choice. There are plenty of opportunities to get involved in stuff during the school year. I did not come from the background of any research or didn't have anything like that on my CV and suddenly in 2nd or 3rd year felt like I needed to have something. It's still pretty thin, but I have a couple of things that I said yes to, and they became things that I could write down on my resume - then talk about even though none of them are complete, none of them are published or anything like that… they're just projects. They are ongoing and may or may not become something concrete in the future, but they are stuff to talk about, stuff to write on your resume, and stuff to talk about during interviews.

## Cameron Smith, Internal Medicine

My first summer off, I lived back home and worked about 30 hours a week in a research laboratory at a local university in the short 8 week break that we had. The work was difficult, and my PI had very high expectations and the job demanded a steep learning curve. In the end, I didn't end up publishing any of my work either. In retrospect, I would have either worked on a simpler project, or would have dedicated half of my summer to working and the other half to just having fun. As they say, the summer after your first year is really the last time when you can potentially have 1-2 months of time off (that is until fourth year). If you are going to work, I think it's really important to do something you find meaningful and that you like!

## Alyssa Mendelson, General Surgery

Do whatever you want with your time off. Some people did nothing, some went to Asia with their fiancés, some did research, some tutored. When it comes down to it, you have enough time during school to "round out" your experience with things like research and publications. If you want a more in-depth project, sure, use your first summer to do some research. If you're exhausted and need to lay on the couch and watch Gilmore Girls or Game of Thrones, do it – and don't let anyone tell you you're being stupid. It's important to take good care of yourself. Medical school is a marathon. Rest if you need to.

Go on an international trip, if possible. It's fun and looks great on your application. I was able to get to Cuba for an "Exploration of the Cuban Healthcare System." Not only was it informative, productive and a great academic experience, but I was able to drink Mojitos and hang out with a couple classmates. And I learned to salsa dance.

Considering I've had like 3 months of fourth year completely off, I'm going to say no. It's your last real "summer," but you certainly get time off at other times.

## Burt Johnson, Urology

Between my first and second year of medical school I had a fantastic experience that was perfect for me. After the first year I needed a little bit of a break, but I wanted to be mildly productive as well. I set up a part-time research project by emailing an urologist, and we started working on a couple projects. The urologist and I communicated very clearly about our expectations. I told him that I was interested in getting something done and being productive, but that a flexible schedule would be preferable. We arranged my work to be very flexible and often could be done remotely. Most importantly I was able to spend the summer with my girlfriend. A bonus was that I established a relationship with someone who is a productive researcher and a supporter of my professional goals. What started out as one publication and a few side projects, turned into great personal and professional relationship.

The other aspect about the summer between first and second year is that it really truly isn't the last summer that you'll ever have. Look forward to 4th year…

## Tyler van Backer, General Surgery

Everyone told me to have a great vacation my summer after first year- that it was my last time off. While it's true that this time is probably the last time I will have a dedicated 8 weeks off in a row, fourth year is right behind it in terms of vacation and responsibilities.

I would not have changed how I spent my time. I put a lot of time into my research and working a job outside of school, which boded well for me when it came to interviews.

## Mairin Jerome, PM & R

What you do with your time off becomes progressively less important as you advance in medical school. I had both a "productive" and fun time during the summer between 1st and 2nd year. Having some significant research experience that you can talk about intelligently during interviews is important.

In my opinion, establishing a research project during the summer between 1st and 2nd year is a great use of your time. I ended up doing a clinical and research surgical month in India with a mission based care organization. There are many global health opportunities out there and most schools have grants or funds students can apply for to help offset the cost. I worked with a center that was collecting vast quantities of patient outcomes data, so not only did I gain surgical experience, but I also did a smaller, initial research project that resulted in 2 poster presentations but also allowed for expansion of the study for the following 2 years to include more patients, which has ultimately resulted in a manuscript submitted for publication with me as first author. Thus, if you can find an interesting project that you are actually excited about, that can lead to both a presentation and a manuscript that you can continue after the summer, this can be very helpful. Travelling somewhere internationally also allows for fun travel time before, during, or after, so you at least have some down time before starting second year.

## Whitney Alduron, Anesthesia

I spent the summer between first and second year doing a research project which was probably the best thing I have ever done. It wasn't a significant amount of time each day and therefore I had plenty of time to travel, hike, swim, play kickball, and hang out with my friends. Yet, it gave me a little bit of direction each day/week and in the end, my work was picked up by one of the pulmonary fellows and resulted in a publication.

I think residency programs like to see well-rounded students who have lives outside of school. Spend time during school (as well as in the summer) doing things that you love and find interesting. It's fun and gives you conversation topics during residency interviews.

One of the best things that you can do (if you know the field you want to pursue) would be to approach a professor/physician and do a research project with them. It can benefit you in so many ways. The most obvious benefits are that it shows initiative, interest, and allows you to develop a relationship with a faculty member who could write you a meaningful letter of recommendation. Any poster, project, or publication that comes out of it is just icing on the cake. Realistically, projects like these can be done over a period of months or years and therefore it is not a significant amount of time and can easily be done in the background of your normal work.

## Harold Callahan, Dermatology

I took the summer of my first year off and had a great time. I also had a solid research background from prior work so I wasn't worried about my CV looking light. If you have a few projects lined up, basically something to put on ERAS and something fun to talk about on the interview trail, you are all set.

Come up with your own project or invention even if it's not in the field you're applying in. Try to have photos or videos of what you did on your phone or a tablet. People like pictures and it breaks up all the talking. They just want to see initiative.

# G. Michael Krauthamer, Emergency Medicine

If you are like me, and took some time off during medical school, you will hear that this will count against you during the residency process. I found the opposite was true. The caveat here is that you should do something interesting during your time off. In my case, I volunteered at a free health clinic for homeless people in Philadelphia. Obviously medical school does not offer much time for extracurriculars, but the volunteer experience helped me hone my professional aspirations, and gave me something interesting to talk about during the interview.

# 6

# CLERKSHIP YEAR

## Calvin Barber, Anesthesia

For clerkship year, if I was smart I would have bought a one year subscription to UWorld Qbank and been doing those all the way through the year because I repeatedly got into honors territory on a clerkship and screwed it up by doing really poorly on the shelf exam. I didn't do enough questions at all during my third year, and very nearly failed a couple of those exams. I got really close to failing Ob/Gyn after having done really well on a rotation and feeling like I knew stuff. For me, I need to get into the zone of multiple choice testing, of recognizing what they are looking for rather than overthinking and picking the red herring which I do invariably.

I hated the fact that all through the pre-clinical years, everyone could theoretically get honors if they attained a certain threshold score, and then as you start clerkships you are competing against most of the people in your clerkship group because only three people can get an honors grade. That just seemed offensive to me. If you want to encourage people to work together, make it so that everyone can honor if they meet criteria.

## Burt Johnson, Urology

Based upon clinical evaluations from faculty and supervising residents, I qualified for honors for most clerkships. My weakness was with my shelf exams. In hindsight I would've at least tried to buy a one-year subscription to UWorld and then do all the corresponding questions during each clerkship. I was able to honor 2 of 7 clerkships. So I'd like to think that with a little bit more dedication to actual reading and doing practice questions, I could've bumped that up. For the best results, you want honor as many clerkships as possible, they actually do appear to matter. They're much more relevant and important to your overall profile than preclinical grades.

In that light, there are definitely students everyone knows that really have a difficult time balancing their academic aspirations with professional collegiality.

> *"While a poor evaluation may not be a big deal, having all of your future professional colleagues remember how you embarrassed them will stick for rest of their lives and they'll remember what an asshole you were."*
>
> -Burt Johnson

Being a gunner seldom benefits you, don't be that person. Your fellow students will not appreciate it. The reality is that while it is cliché that med school is a marathon, it is true and eventually it will come back and bite you in the ass. Just like the scene from Good Will Hunting where the Harvard barney embarrasses Ben Affleck in the bar in front of some ladies, listen to Matt Damon and take his life lesson to never embarrass someone to make yourself look good, particularly if it's your classmate. If there's one thing that attending physicians and residents despise, it's throwing your colleagues under the bus. While a poor evaluation may not be a big deal, having all of your future professional colleagues remember how you embarrassed them will stick for rest of their lives and they'll remember what an asshole you were. So for everyone's sake, don't do that.

Scheduling clerkships - evaluate what specialties you're interested in. When I started clerkship year I had a fairly good idea that I would want to do surgery or pediatrics. I chose to do surgery as my third clerkship and pediatrics was my last, just because that's how the rotations were ordered at my school. I felt it was more important to recognize that I wanted to do a surgical specialty early so that I could prepare for fourth-year scheduling and get away rotations set up. I thought because pediatrics was a little less competitive, if I did it last and fell in love with it, I could throw things together pretty quickly for that application process.

I think the optimal spot for your clerkship(s) of interest is anywhere, but at the end of your clerkship year. If you do your specialty of interest first or second, it's totally fine because expectations are low and your energy level will be high. Doing your clerkship of interest somewhere in the middle works because you will know the ropes of how the hospital runs. You can focus your energy on actually participating in care, learning about the specialty, and demonstrating your attitude, aptitude, and interest. This also affords you enough time to get things set up afterward for your fourth-year.

A downside of doing a clerkship somewhere in the middle is that this is also the conventional wisdom on scheduling your clerkship year, so if you're interested in surgery, for example, you will probably be in a group with other motivated people who want to do surgery. This will make it more difficult to honor surgery or other clerkships for that matter, because surgery seems to attract competitive people. Doing your clerkship of interest at the end of your third year poses a challenge. It can be logistically more challenging to arrange your fourth-year, but you can make it work if need be.

## Samuel Austin, Anesthesia

Looking back on clerkship year I think I wouldn't have taken it so seriously in the beginning. By your fourth or fifth rotation you start feeling pretty comfortable in your role as a clinical clerk. In truth, there were days early on when I had to tell myself that "you just need to show up" in order to get out of bed. Later on I came to realize that Shelf exams are just another test and that the ACGME requirements for each rotation were more often than not useless generators of stress. What made my year and has colored the rest of my journey through medical school? Coming back to the notion that caring for patients is an absolute privilege. Whether you realize it or not, you will – or have – emulated many of the people you worked with in third year. Mirror the good traits you see in residents, attendings, nurses, environmental staff, and your fellow students. There are wonderful people everywhere you look that you can learn from if you are aware enough to appreciate their lessons. Don't let a shitty resident or attending take away from the experience.

Don't be a dick to your classmates. Some of my best from medical school friends were in my flight group.

## Harold Cunningham, Dermatology

No matter where you go to school, or which hospital you rotate at, these grades can be very hard to control as they are inherently subjective. Clerkship and Residency Directors know this, but they expect you to honor some of them and have solid comments in all of them. This is also heavily dependent on the school you attend and what their percentage of students honor per clerkship. The percentage of honors given varies between 20-60% depending on the school and clerkship. Schools may think they are adding value to the grade by only awarding a low percentage of honors, but more often than not, this can theoretically penalize a larger number of students. Clerkship grades are another box that can be checked on ERAS (and potentially used as a filter).

## Whitney Alduron, Anesthesiology

Obviously clerkships at different schools are all slightly different but I wish that I had known going into it that I would be graded against members of my clerkship (flight) group. I chose a flight group that was predominantly made up of my friends. Unfortunately all of my friends are smart, hardworking, outgoing, charismatic, personable, well liked individuals and that was reflected in the difficulty of honoring clerkships. I ended up not honoring any clerkships and I felt that was not a reflection of me, but a reflection of the competitiveness of my flight group. This is very difficult/impossible to justify without sounding whiny. It would have been nice to know ahead of time how the grading worked within the clerkship groups and whether you are graded against your peers in your flight group or against your peers in your class as a whole.

> *"The best way to do well is to be your genuine self, so long as your genuine self is a caring, empathic, interested, motivated, intelligent, on-the-ball, caffeinated third year medical student who is going into the specialty you're currently rotating through."*
>
> *-Samuel Austin*

## Cameron Smith, Internal Medicine

I started clerkship year much more timid than I am now. There were times when I felt like a burden on the residents, fellows, and attendings with whom I was working, and so I would avoid asking questions. Eventually, I had the realization that I was there to learn and staying quiet when I had a question didn't help my learning experience or my grade. It's definitely important to feel out situations and ask questions when the time is appropriate. However, if you do have a question at an inopportune time, save it and ask it later. Being excessively eager can seem disingenuous, but again, staying silent shows that you're just not interested.

The advice I give to third-years is to fully immerse yourself in every rotation. Even if you know that you're not going into that specialty, pretend for that rotation that you're a future neurologist, psychiatrist, surgeon etc.. That way, you'll stay fascinated by the material and get the most out of your time instead of wallowing in your misery.

Grades definitely matter in your clerkship year, but again, they are only one piece of the pie. Do your best to honor every rotation that you can, while remembering to save enough time to study for the shelf exams. However, after a rotation is over, don't beat yourself up about a sub-par grade. Move on and do your best on the next rotation.

> *"What made my clerkship year and has colored the rest of my journey through medical school? Coming back to the notion that caring for patients is an absolute privilege."*
>
> -Samuel Austin

My only advice regarding scheduling your clerkships is not to have your first rotation be the specialty that you want to go into. Even if you have a remote possibility of entering that field, try not to do it until the third or fourth rotation. That way, you have the experience of what it's like to be a third-year, and can give it your all.

## Alyssa Mendelson, General Surgery

Prior to scheduling clerkships, I did not know that I wanted to be a general surgeon. I did my Surgery clerkship first and I've heard people recommend that you do it later in the year so you're "smarter on the wards." Honestly, I don't think it mattered. I worked my ass off, I was enthusiastic about learning, and that's really all residents and attendings could ask for. They didn't care that I knew nothing (literally nothing), they cared about my attitude and how much I improved. I ended up honoring my clerkship even though that was my lowest shelf score throughout 3rd year. Wherever you end up putting them, just do your best and be a fun person to work with.

Yes, grades matter here too. Again, if you are going into a competitive specialty, at least try to honor the "big" clerkships – Surgery or Internal Medicine. If you know you want to go into Surgery, try to honor that clerkship. Same goes for the other specialties. If you don't honor them, don't sweat it too much. Again, I know people who honored none or only one clerkship and they are still applying to competitive specialties. If you're passionate enough, I think it can be done!

## Whitney Alduron, Anesthesia

I think etiquette to fellow classmates is extremely important, and I believe my school has an excellent culture of camaraderie and cooperativeness. I never felt as though I was being stepped on by my classmates or thrown under the bus, and I would never think to do that to others. In the long run, we are all going to be physicians and coworkers and no one will remember who honored and who didn't, but people will remember who treated them like shit and stepped on them to get ahead.

Rotations at satellite hospitals were tricky because sometimes you had absolutely no idea what to expect, and I think you just need to be ready to roll with the punches and fall in with the culture of the hospital. For us, a lot of the away rotations were not at "teaching hospitals" which meant the attitudes and culture at the hospital could be very different. Without medical students around on a daily basis, I felt as though physicians forget how little you know, and it can sometimes be very discouraging.

For anesthesia, clerkship order does not matter because it is not one of the clerkship specialties. However, I think that it is probably important if you want to go into a clerkship specialty (i.e. neurology, OB, surgery) to have it placed in the middle of the year. That way, you know enough that you don't look like a total idiot, but it's not at the end of the year where you are tired and burned out. I can safely say that anesthesia residency programs don't care how well you do in other specialties during your clerkship year because it has relatively little to do with how well you will perform as an anesthesia resident.

## Tyler van Backer, General Surgery

I did surgery third. If you can only get your prized clerkship first or last, it's most certainly not the end of the world. If you have a choice, I found it helpful to have a couple of rotations under my belt so I knew simple things already (i.e. what a postop note is, how to use the EMR, how to present patients, etc.). I did not honor my surgery clerkship and no one said anything about it, but my MSPE comments were very favorable from the Clerkship Director, so it's not 100% you must honor the rotation. Obviously, it's important to try and better if you do, though.

Grades matter for surgery. You can match having not honored a rotation, but the more "Hs" on your transcript, the better, assuming that the comments that go in the MSPE reflect this (i.e. don't disappear from clinical duties to just go study to ace the shelf... this will reflect poorly on your overall evaluation if staff don't feel like you care at all about the rotation).

Remember, your classmates are your colleagues. Treat them with the same respect you would if they were evaluating you. Throwing other students under the bus to make yourself look better is easy for attendings and residents to see through. Rotations can be hard enough without having an obnoxious gunner trying to show off.

## Mairin Jerome, PM & R

I would have used questions banks/book more for studying for the shelf exams. I also did not know the NBME publishes practice shelf exams. One thing I did realize towards the end of the year is that it is okay to take care of yourself if you have doctor's appointments or things you need to do. It's okay to ask. During my first few rotations I felt like I had to be there no matter what, but it is okay if you are sick to not come in.

Don't be an asshole to your fellow classmates (or anyone, for that matter). Be helpful, share information, be pleasant and courteous to those around you. Be nice and respectful to nurses - they know a lot more than you at this stage. Grades are important during clerkships. Residency programs are getting so many applications that they are beginning to use honoring that specialty's clerkship as a screening tool.

I had the benefit of doing a year-long pathology fellowship between my 3rd and 4th years. I was evaluated based on my clinical performance during this year and had mostly honors for each rotation which benefitted me.

# 7

# THE OUTSIDE WORLD

*Extracurriculars, Service, and Research*

*Was it important for the application process? Perhaps it mattered more in life? Drew from it to formulate personal statement?*

## Burt Johnson, Urology

It's difficult to decipher what was important from this particular category. During medical school I was involved with an organization that provides a mobile health clinic with free healthcare to rural villages and country in Africa. I was the point person in the United States for projects, and it was something that was important to me, and I also thought that residency programs might think it's interesting. Perhaps they did when they read my application on paper, however I was never asked about it. I would suspect that this is very specialty dependent.

An additional item that is something Harold mentioned, our fellow contributing author who applied to dermatology. He said something of particular interest which resonated with me and that was to invent or create something. During medical school, I worked on a few medical device projects and a software project. I was asked about these projects at every single interview. I anticipated this and brought a small tablet with me to show pictures of all my professional work. This was a huge asset for me when it came to interviews. Do I think it was particularly important or stood out on my paper application? Maybe it was because it was listed under a patent, but it could have been glossed over easily. The theme is being creative, pursuing your idea, and pursuing it with a passion. That's what program directors care about. Find a way to stand out from the herd.

## Calvin Barber, Anesthesia

I did a lot of volunteering before medical school and nobody asked me about stuff I did in the fourth year. In the fourth year, I went away to Guatemala for a month, but it was late in the year so I was doing interviews as I was preparing to go - so nobody asked about it.

Before medical school, I raised money for UNICEF and stuff like that, several people asked about that, and I think it was important, but more so when it came to getting into medical school in the first place. The interviews to get into medical school were a completely different set of interviews compared to those of residency. The residency interviews were really nice, and I liked them a lot, and felt welcomed and wanted. Interviews for medical school were a whole different kettle of fish.

*"How obnoxious is the person in your class that literally ONLY has medicine? You invite them out to dinner and all they talk about are tests, clerkships, etc. How many times have you wanted to kill that person?"*

*-Alyssa Mendelson*

I think having a particular rotation that you really enjoyed and can talk about - I think is useful and important. Giving the impression that you actually like medicine, that you like the specialty that you are trying to match into, that you like other specialties as well, I think all those things come off in a positive way. If you are in an interview and you seem excited and positive and happy with your life, it makes you really appealing.

## Alyssa Mendelson, General Surgery

Do extracurriculars. Not just because it rounds out your application, but because it keeps you human during medical school. If your entire life is medical school, you are going to lose sight of a lot of important things in life, and likely you're going to be very boring to talk to and work with. Don't be the person who does a million things because it looks great on an application, choose a few things you truly love to do and try to maintain them during school.

I love field hockey – I played in college and didn't want to give it up during medical school. So, I joined an adult league and played for all four years of medical school. I also was able to pick up an assistant coaching position for a high school varsity field hockey team in my second and fourth year of medical school. These things made me SO MUCH happier, and they made nice conversations during my interviews!

> *"I was involved in a lot of interest groups and I did a Schweitzer Fellowship project. In hindsight, I am not sure if this was the best use of my time."*
>
> *-Mairin Jerome*

Seriously, just have some interests outside of medical school. No one cares what they are, as long as you're passionate about them. How obnoxious is the person in your class that literally ONLY has medicine? You invite them out to dinner and all they talk about are tests, clerkships, etc. How many times have you wanted to kill that person? That's probably how your interviewers are going to feel too…

## Harold Cunningham, Dermatology

Important all around. I recommend doing a lot of different volunteer activities and adventures. The more obscure the better. You need to fill a lot of space on that ERAS CV and having random cool things to talk about is what people remember. They don't want to talk about your research.

They use your activities outside the hospital to try to figure out what type of person you are and if you will be a good fit in the program and area. If you talk about how much love skiing then programs in Florida will do you a favor by not interviewing you.

## Cameron Smith, Internal Medicine

Extracurriculars can only help. The most important thing is to spend time on activities that you value. If you're doing stuff just to put on your CV, it's easy to tell and comes off as again as disingenuous during interviews. The content of the extracurriculars doesn't really matter, just that you're able to speak passionately about what interested you, and demonstrate that you were able to be passionate about something and bring it to completion.

## Tyler van Backer, General Surgery

The extracurricular activities you do are certainly important. Residencies want to see that you're more than just a medical student who studies in the library. You don't have to be leading medical expeditions to under-served populations in Africa (although, kudos if you do). Playing in an intramural sports league, having a musical hobby, or writing a cookbook are all good stress reliefs and show you're well-rounded. Residency will be challenging and programs want to know that you have the coping mechanisms and are able to deal with stress in a healthy manner. Few things look worse than a high attrition rate for future applicants to a program.

As touched on above, programs really want to see that you're a real person and have coping strategies. If you drop out of a residency, it looks really bad for them, so they have a vested interest in keeping their residents (in addition to wanting to train competent doctors). Depending what residency you're considering, you'll also be there for anywhere from 3-7+ years, so programs want to also have a vague idea if you'll fit in (i.e. are all your hobbies related to a big city, yet the program is located in a rural setting).

As an example, I work on an ambulance and had several interviewers who also worked as EMTs prior to residency, so it was a nice bonding point. Residents, though, didn't review the file unless they were interviewing me, so that was more informal and they seemed to genuinely just want to know what I did for fun. Having a commonality also makes it easier to remind interviewers about your conversation and therefore who you were when/if you send thank you cards.

## Whitney Alduron, Anesthesia

I personally did not do any volunteer activities during medical school. With regards to extracurricular activities, I think it is more important to have some as opposed to what they actually are. In almost all of my residency interviews, the interviewer asked about an extracurricular activity I had listed on my application. It was definitely a talking point and often interviewers would pick up on something we had in common, and it would make the conversations easier. Although I have to admit my roommate listed "catching up on the latest TV shows" as an extracurricular activity and people seem to actually enjoy/connect with that. So anything you write down is better than nothing apparently.

# Research

## Calvin Barber, Anesthesia

I managed to get a whole bunch of things on my CV down as research that, strictly speaking, were not 'completed' projects. I haven't published anything, never claimed to have published anything, but I have been involved with several research projects. Back in September, I had several things that I was planning to do as research projects, some of which are alive and well, and maybe will be finished one day, and some which may never turn into anything. I think it's absolutely fair game to put everything down on your resume, your application, but be prepared to say, "yeah ultimately I didn't get IRB approval for that, or that didn't work" or have some kind of story for the things you didn't do, if you're comfortable with that.

## Hank Ng, Internal Medicine

I really do think if you go into certain specialties, you need to do research or get involved in that field before application season. I think all my orthopedic friends did some research either in the first two classroom years or at least by third year. The same thing happened for urology. No one did ophthalmology in our class, but I assume the same rule applies.

As for myself, I thought I would have an interest in hematology/oncology and tried to get involved in research, but couldn't find anything initially. I am sure if I pushed I could have found something – I ended up doing some work in 4th year. If you find yourself in this position, one of my classmates actually started up a research relationship with a different academic medical institution that had a greater emphasis on research.

I did outside activities I valued. I am a big runner and joined our marathon team. I love soccer, and I organized pick up soccer and played some intramurals. I just chose activities I valued: helping refugees learn about our health care system, teaching kids about human anatomy and medicine, helping out some friends with their own projects. I didn't lead any groups or publish a paper, I didn't do a poster presentation or lead any committees, and I didn't do any research until my third year. On my interviews they were pretty general about my extracurriculars – they ranged from asking me about stuff all the way back in high school until what I had done most recently. Whatever was on ERAS was fair game, but they were always nice about everything. Mainly superficial open ended questions like, "tell me more about building the bridge, or refugee health, public health project, or undergraduate research." It was never really mean stuff – nothing like "oh you did research on this, do you know the most current guidelines or most up to date research in the field now?"

## Tyler van Backer, General Surgery

For surgical specialties, it is important to have research. If you can, set up a research project and really take charge, showing residency programs that you show initiative, leadership, and interest. If you're not very interested in research, that is okay, too. Taking charge and orchestrating something you're passionate about is good as well.

Several programs that I interviewed at are starting to require research papers during residency, even if residents don't get protected research time, and others had defined research requirements. Showing that you have experience with the process can be a selling point for you, especially if you took the lead on a project, wrote the IRB, won a grant, etc.

Another piece of advice I can give is to keep your CV updated as you go along in medical school. It's much easier to just jot items down as you go along rather than trying to remember everything at the last minute, you will inevitably miss things.

## G. Michael Krauthamer, Emergency Medicine

With regard to research experience: If you are like me (and many medical students are) you will have done some research prior to or during medical school. If so, emphasize it. My application appealed to academic programs, and the bulk of my interview invitations reflected this. During interviews, I made sure to emphasize my interest in academic medicine to further punctuate my suitability for these programs.

When relevant, I made sure to discuss areas of research and education that continue to interest me, and ideas I had for pursuing these while in residency.

If you are one of those students who has limited or no research experience, consider allotting time early in your fourth year to work on a project or poster for presentation that you can include on your application.

## Mairin Jerome, PM & R

Research is important for developing your own critical thinking skills as an investigator, but can also be an asset when it comes time for residency applications.

## Samuel Austin, Anesthesia

Research is actually a pretty great thing, and I think most people can find a project that is personally satisfying and interesting. Programs are generally interested in research. It is a great way to demonstrate interest in your chosen specialty, to get to know the players at your home institution, and to appreciate the direction that your field is going in.

## Alyssa Mendelson, General Surgery

If you are applying to high-powered academic programs (in general surgery), you need to have research. They will all want to see this and will want you to talk about it.

## Whitney Alduron, Anesthesia

I ended up with strong research component on my application, and I was asked about it at every interview more or less. The research experience helped me get interviews at more academic programs because anesthesia is not traditionally a research heavy field, and they are eager to attract candidates who would like to pursue research in the future. However, it was just a lucky coincidence that the research ended up benefiting me because I never did research for the purpose of bolstering my application.

# Volunteering

## Alyssa Mendelson, General Surgery

I did a couple, not because I wanted to improve my application but because opportunities presented themselves and they frankly were fun. My two big volunteering activities were at the annual Breast Care Conference and the Girl's Science Discovery Day. Both were a chance to give back in areas where I had both professional and personal interest.

## Mairin Jerome, PM & R

My background prior to medical school and during was very strong with regards to volunteer experience, particularly international and underserved populations.

In first and second year, I was involved in a lot of interest groups and I did a Schweitzer Fellowship project. In hindsight, I am not sure if this was the best use of my time. It was helpful to be able to talk about this, but medical school is tough academically, particularly for a non-traditional applicant with a background in art.

In hindsight, my time would have been spent more wisely during the first 2 years just studying and doing as well as I could academically (ultimately in preparation for Step 1). I still had enough experiences to talk about from before med school and the summer between first and second year.

# 8

# 4TH YEAR AND AWAY ROTATIONS

*Impression and General Experiences*

## Calvin Barber, Anesthesiology

Because of the specific requirements, I thought doing away rotations was likely to be very significant for me, very important - for me to be taken seriously as a strong candidate. As I've said before I don't have standout board scores (236 Step 1), I don't have a series of pre-clinical or clerkship courses that I honored, so I thought doing an away rotation would be helpful. I tried to set up four away rotations in total, two of which actually came to fruition. In both of the places I did away rotations, I got interviews and feel very strongly that they liked me very much and ranked me highly. So for my specific circumstances, I really think doing an away rotation was critical to my chances of getting a residency position.

It's hard to shake the feeling that I might not have been interviewed at the two places where I did away rotations, but it's possibly true. In terms of doing an away rotation, one of the places that I rotated, the chief of anesthesia said to me in no uncertain terms, "You need to do really well while you're here. Your application may be strong, may be weak, doesn't matter. It has nothing like the power of how you do when you are here with us for a month."

I think that that is so clearly true. If any program ever says to you that being there for a month doesn't influence them, they are being disingenuous. So I kind of appreciated the bluntness, disturbing though it was, and there was a little hint of implied intimidation as this was early in my rotation. I appreciated the 'clarity' shall we say.

> *"If you think that doing well on a rotation at a big-name center will help you match there, I have bad news, at least in Derm. Odds are you will never meet the chair or director, let alone work with them."*
>
> -Harold Callahan

I did not ever seek to do an away rotation with the intention of getting a letter from recommendation from that program. I think that wasn't relevant for me. I think if you go to a program to do an away rotation, your goal is to impress them with what a fun person you are to have around. Perhaps to show them you're smart as well, but not everyone has the capacity to do that. For anesthesia, I don't think that it's as important to impress with knowledge, it's not as important as being a nice person to have around. Again if we're talking about why I think I matched to anesthesia at a specific program, I think it's due to spending a month there and simply being nice. Being really interested in stuff, genuinely interested in stuff - that's another pearl of wisdom, never fake it. Personally, I never fake it. If I'm interested in something, I engage and certainly try to show how interested I am, but I never fake it. Being at an institution for a month, it is so much about whether you are, in anesthesia particularly where you spend a lot of time in conversation, it's about whether you are going to be the kind of person that I want to be hanging out with at 3 AM.

Do I trust that you are competent? Do you do stupid weird stuff? Are you some kind of freak and I didn't it pick it up from your application? Or do you have some good stories to tell and are kind of cool to hang out with? I think that's why matched at a great program.

If you know what you're going to apply to, I knew I'd do anesthesia, you should do an anesthesia month at your own institution before you do an away rotation, if your home institution has a residency program. It would be a mistake to go do a month of anesthesia at a place you are hoping to match at if you have not been through a month at your own, friendly institution.

At my home program, the program director flat out said he always is concerned about an applicant who couldn't honor the specialty at their home program. This naturally puts pressure on the program to honor their own students. If you want to do surgery, they know you want to do surgery, and they don't give you honors for doing a fourth year rotation, they're saying, "we are going to cause you problems," and they know they're saying it. So do you have to honor your own institution? Yeah I think you do.

## Samuel Austin, Anesthesia

Fourth year rotations are absolutely crucial in my opinion. I was between several specialties in the beginning of my fourth year (orthopedics, EM, and anesthesiology). It took doing a rotation in each before I felt absolutely sure in my decision to pursue anesthesiology, as it reminded me of all the reasons why I went to medical school (chief amongst those reasons is to become better at Sudoku).

I also did an away rotation in anesthesiology at UCSF. It is by no means necessary to do away rotations, at least in anesthesiology, but it helped me get an idea of the type of program I wanted to train at. I was floored by the complex and high-stakes procedures at UCSF and felt intimidated, but also inspired, by the extremely bright residents and faculty. I was able to get a letter from them, and it most certainly helped my application and gave me confidence that I could pass for a fourth year medical student in places other than my home institution. Not only that, but it was a blast to go to another city and meet people. I'm still in close contact with another visiting student with whom I rotated. See, reader? Your mom was right: you'll make friends everywhere you go.

Medicine is regional in the way it's practiced. Away rotations are helpful in most areas, but talk with your advisor if you're unsure. Do a rotation at your home institution before doing an away if you can. It is a good way to get polished to impress people and feel less intimidated when visiting another hospital.

## Whitney Alduron, Anesthesia

I did an away rotation at the University of Utah in November. The only benefit to doing and away after July is to get better insight into a specific program. Since it was after the application due date, I did not get any letters of recommendation and my grade did not count on my application. It is definitely not necessary to do away rotations for anesthesia, but Utah was a place I was highly considering for residency and so I wanted to get a closer look.

Also I feel that doing an away rotation almost guarantees you an interview at a place they may not have considered you before, especially for geographic reasons.

> *"You need to do really well while you're here. Your application may be strong, may be weak, doesn't matter. It has nothing like the power of how you do when you are here with us for a month."*
>
> **-Program Director**

The University of Utah interviewed me during my rotation, but it also happened to be during interview season. I ran into other students who had done aways at Utah and had to return for the official interview during November/December. They did not offer a less formal interview during their away rotation. Doing an away rotation made the interview process very easy. I felt as though they almost treated me like a "home" student in the sense that they had gotten a chance to know me, and we could have a normal conversation as opposed to peppering me with questions about my application. It also gave me a chance to gush about how much I really liked the program, and that it was a top choice of mine for residency without sounding empty or meaningless. Coming all the way out from the East coast to spend a month makes the impression that you're serious about a program in a very direct way.

I honestly recommend doing at least one away rotation at the program you think is a top choice for residency. My opinion is that it definitely feels like it gives you a significant advantage over other students in a specialty where away rotations are not required or even encouraged. Doing an away rotation is useful if you are interested in going somewhere for residency that you have never been before and have no connections to. That being said you need to prioritize and only pick one or possibly two locations to go to because away rotations are exhausting and costly.

## Tyler van Backer, General Surgery

My first rotation was an away. I would not suggest it. I still interviewed at the place where I did my first AI/Sub-I, but I wish I had more time to work out the kinks/understand my role better as a fourth year. However, the upside was that I was much sharper and prepared for my home rotation, the source of my recommendation letters.

To prepare for a general surgery away month, I tried to read about common problems (e.g. bowel obstructions, appendectomies, cholecystectomies, etc.) and be comfortable with post-operative management and H&Ps. Enthusiasm and a willingness to help out are fundamental qualities that residents and attendings are looking for at most institutions. On a preparation-related note, knowing your patients inside and out and any patient you see in the OR is expected. Attendings will notice if you're on the ball and can answer questions about a patient's post-operative course. Likewise, if you go into a case and don't know what's going on, that will not reflect poorly on you, but that's pretty obvious.

The importance of away rotations is somewhat debated. The "pro-away" camp, like me, think that it's an excellent way to show off your skills and see a program for more than 8 hours (interview day), where anyone can put up a front. It's hard to hide unhappy residents, malignant attendings, and other bothers for an entire month. If you work your hardest and get along with the residents, that speaks volumes. It also gives you an opportunity to see what life would be like living in that city or area. For me, it was very important because my boards were good, but I wasn't AOA and I wanted to try to interview at some of the more competitive programs, as well. I also felt like I wasn't sure whether I wanted a purely academic or community based program, or somewhat of a mix, so it was good to see the difference, first-hand and get a feel for what fit my learning style better. The "against-away" camp argues that it can really hurt you if you mess up or piss off the wrong person, which is also certainly true.

I met with the program director and chair at one place, but did not interview there. I certainly felt like I knew the programs and residents I rotated with more than the ones I just interviewed at for eight hours.

## Cameron Smith, Internal Medicine

Certain faculty at my home institution advised me that doing away rotations at places where I can see myself doing internal medicine residency was not necessary, and wouldn't really benefit me. I was told that this would benefit those going into smaller fields, like urology or dermatology, but wouldn't really benefit someone going into internal medicine. This couldn't have been farther from the truth.

I did three away rotations at places where I thought I would be interested in residency training. The opportunity gave me the ability to "feel out" different programs and get an idea of the culture at different institutions. It also gave me the ability to go to places where I was interested, work hard, and demonstrate that I would be both a good resident and someone that is excited to be there. If you do away rotations with the mentality that you will work hard and demonstrate your abilities, I think they can only help. You may even be able to sit down with the program director during the end of some of your away rotations and demonstrate your interest and what attributes you liked about that program.

I received an interview at every center at which I did an away rotation. Whether or not the interviews invitations were based on my application or my evaluations during the rotation, I don't know. Regardless, the away rotations only helped. Every site I rotated at brought me back for a scheduled interview day rather than a formal interview at the conclusion of my away month. I felt like the rotation gave me an opportunity to discuss with my interviewer attributes of the program that I liked, as well as individual attendings with whom I enjoyed working. This can go a long way.

## Alyssa Mendelson, General Surgery

I didn't do any! And literally no one cared. Apparently it's not that important in Surgery.

## Harold Callahan, Dermatology

I have a home program in dermatology. I did two away rotations at large, big-name hospitals because I had friends that lived in the cities. In hindsight, this is not how you want to arrange away rotations. Away rotations can be very useful and at the very least should guarantee you an interview and a  high ranking. If you go to a big place this will not be the case in dermatology. They don't care that you are there for a month, and wrote a case report – and they don't want to write you a letter.

Your best bet is to go to a smaller, more rural program for away rotations. Use doximity's server to find the email for the program coordinator and ask what months they have open, if the chair and director will be there (they do go on vacation), and if you will work directly with them. If the answers are yes, then go. Then you can ask the chair and/or director for a meaningful letter because you worked with them. Remember letters from chairs and directors have their own little boxes to check off on the ERAS! If the answers are no then don't waste your time.

I know you will have to rent a place and the program won't be a big name, but your chances of matching are greatly increased. And frankly, in Dermatology, that's what it's all about. If you think that doing well on a rotation at a big-name center will help you match there, I have bad news. Odds are you will never meet the chair or director, let alone work with them. Which means that a meaningful letter is out of the question. If they are a research program, they probably have students that took a year off and are conducting research there already. Those students plus the home institution students make it pretty hard for a chair/director to justify writing a letter for someone they never worked with and was there for only one month. Honestly, you may not even get an interview.

One away gave me an interview, and another did not (despite two letters from faculty, a case report, and presenting at ground rounds).

What you should generate from an away rotation is an interview, at the very least. If you don't, then you planned it poorly. In Dermatology, there is no end of the month interview stuff. If they want you, then you have to come back in December and January for formal interviews. Unless you are doing your away at that time, you will be traveling again.

## Burt Johnson, Urology

Selecting away rotations was a thoughtful process. In hindsight after interviewing, doing two away rotations, and meeting many people on the interview trail who spent time doing rotations at a variety of programs both geographically and in size, structure and culture, I feel like I have much better understanding of how I would select an away rotation, particularly in urology. Sorry for the long sentence.

*"I felt absolutely sure in my decision to pursue anesthesiology, as it reminded me of all the reasons why I went to medical school (chief amongst those reasons is to become better at Sudoku)."*

*-Samuel Austin*

My personal situation was that I wanted to geographically be in New England or the mid-Atlantic and so I targeted programs in Boston. My main criterion was geography – where my girlfriend and I would be happy. I did an away rotation at Boston Medical Center and Massachusetts General Hospital. I wouldn't necessarily recommend doing two away rotations in the same city, but in my personal situation, I was willing to put my eggs into one basket. It wasn't the right time in my life to move to California, despite loving California, Boston or New York were a better fit for next five or six years of my life. It's important to evaluate what your honest desires are for the duration of your training.

Let's say that I had no preference for geography for argument's sake. I would've selected away rotations differently. I specifically got fewer interviewer offers from particular geographic areas, namely California, Pacific Northwest, and the Midwest because I didn't demonstrate any extra interest in those regions, save for sending them my application. Given that I grew up in New England, was student at a medical school in New England, and I did two away rotations in Boston, that all signified to programs that I wanted to stay in the Northeast or the mid-Atlantic. There are so many qualified applicants for so few spots in Urology and other competitive fields that it's very difficult to distinguishing between candidates. I discussed this with many of my co-applicants on the interview trail that the reality is you know roughly 70% of applicants are great candidates. Maybe you can exclude 30%, but you still have 70% and you only have room for a total of 10% of the applicants - at least to invite for an interview. From an academic standpoint, the applicants are roughly on the same level. The reality is programs need to gauge how interested applicants are in their program. I don't think that's any secret. If you're from a particular region and you have no connections to any other region, away rotations are your opportunity to make that connection to another region.

The best way I know to find out information about programs prior to selecting away rotations is to speak with as many people as you can. The best people to talk to are recent applicants who have just gone through the interview process, other residents at your program, and your academic advisors and faculty. The closer someone is to the application process, the more familiar they will be. You want to find out everything about programs from all angles as if you have to make your rank list before you do away rotations. Doing your due diligence will save you from wasting a valuable month and allow you to put yourself in the best position when match day rolls around.

Selecting the proper fourth year away rotations is an underappreciated opportunity. It is a way to prove your worth, demonstrate your geographic interest, and evaluate a program from within. For example, in urology there were many applicants I spoke with who did not do an away rotation in the Midwest and none of them got interviews at any of the Chicago programs. This may be an anomaly and I did not speak with all the applicants, but it was almost common knowledge by the end of interview season that if you wanted a shot at going to a Chicago program, you needed to be connected to them in some way. For programs, it makes sense.

They logistically can't interview every candidate that looks good on paper, so they do their best to figure out who's interested in living in Chicago for five or six years. Understand that fourth-year rotations are opportunities to include yourself in certain groups you may not have belonged to before.

The other vital aspect of an away rotation and fourth-year is experiencing a month at a program. One month out of program can tell you much more about the day-to-day dynamics, training, teaching, surgical experience than one interview day, a day where the program is putting on its best face. One month at a program will never tell you as much as one year or five years at the program, but at some point you'll just have to take the leap anyway.

I wish I had talked to more residents both about their own programs and about programs they visited during their application process. I felt bashful about asking about that stuff while I was on my fourth-year rotations, as I felt like I was partly trying to impress them and make sure they knew I was interested in their program. Don't be bashful. It's important for you to make the right decision for you and not just to try and impress other people.

## G. Michael Krauthamer, Emergency Medicine

While I had rotated in the ED at my school, we do not have a residency program. Thus, I had to schedule a second EM sub-internship at an away program both to secure a SLOE, and because, as I learned from my school advisor, most EM residency programs want applicants who have rotated away from their home institutions. Apparently, residency program directors feel that successfully completing an away sub-internship demonstrates a student's ability to function in the "real-world" of emergency medicine. More importantly, this added experience exposed me to a breadth of EM practice, and provided additional experience to draw on during interviews.

## Jennifer Tango, Emergency Medicine

Setting up fourth year away rotations is extremely important if you are interested in matching at a certain place or venturing to a different region than that of your medical school. It is especially critical if you are coming from a school that does not have a residency program in your specialty. You need to apply for away rotations as early as possible, as spots fill up quickly. If you have a specific place in mind, apply early to get a rotation there. If you want to do residency in a different US region than your school, you should do a rotation in the region you're interested in. I got several interviews because I rotated in a particular region. Program directors recognized one of my letter-writers was from one of my away rotations, and trusted his evaluation. Also, you need to find resources if your school doesn't have a residency program in a particular specialty. Find people who are involved in residency applications/residency education and trust less what people from your school are saying. They very well may have your best interest in mind, but they may not know simply because it's not part of what they regularly do.

## Mairin Jerome, PM & R

I chose not to do a PM & R rotation at my home hospital because they do not have a residency program. Instead, I used some vacation time during my pathology fellowship year to shadow one PM & R doc at my home hospital and one in my hometown. Once I realized I was interested, I set up an away rotation at an academic institution with a strong residency program very early in my 4th year. I ultimately got a letter from the inpatient attending with whom I worked, and I was offered an interview at this program during interview season. Additionally, I obtained a letter from the attending I shadowed from my hometown, who also happens to be on faculty at another strong academic program. Subsequently, I was also offered an interview at this program. If I didn't have this additional letter from the attending I shadowed, it would have been prudent to do another PM & R rotation to get a letter (I think it is optimal to have at least 2 from the field to which you are applying).

It is difficult to determine whether or not I would have been offered interviews at these 2 institutions without rotating there and/or getting a letter from a faculty member. From what I understand, applications to PM & R greatly increased this season, and I was not offered interviews at all of the top programs, presumably because of my scores on Step 1, though I can't know for sure. However, I was offered some interviews at top programs without having connections or having someone call on my behalf.

Either way, if you are interested in a particular program, it is best to err on the side of going there for an away rotation. During interviews, I had some questions about only doing one PM & R rotation. Honestly, for me, it is stressful to move to a different city for a month and get used to a whole new hospital system as a medical student. It didn't seem necessary once I had made up my mind, though probably would have opened more doors to certain programs that were more competitive.

# 9

# ERAS APPLICATION SYSTEM
*The Personal Statement, Deadlines,*
*and Letters of Recommendation*

# The Personal Statement

## Alyssa Mendelson, General Surgery

I hated writing my personal statement. However, it came up as an impressive and important part of my application during interviews, so I'm glad I took the time to make it perfect. Honestly, I really struggled with starting it. Once I had something down on paper it got easier. Initially, I stared at a blank computer screen for hours.

The one thing that got me on track (and please don't judge me for this) was drinking three glasses of wine and just typing whatever came to mind. The next morning I woke up and read what I wrote down and was like "wow, that was super honest." The grammar sucks, but I can use this part and add in blah blah blah. I don't know how it worked, but it did. I guess it made me stop worrying about what I needed to say and phrasing everything just right, and just writing from the heart.

After I wrote my first draft, I sent it to a bunch of people looking for feedback. This was a mistake. I had like six people email me back with their corrections/suggestions, and it was so overwhelming because everyone had a different opinion. Eventually I picked two people as my "I like your suggestions best" people and told the other ones that I appreciate their input, but I'm going another direction. Working with just two people was perfect. Their input was key – you definitely need people from an objective point of view to look at your statement and point out the highlights and what might be missing.

Unless you're a professional poet or something, I'd say stick to something that won't scare program directors…I've heard a lot of people say a great personal statement can't really help your application if it's lacking in other ways, but a bad/weird personal statement can kill an otherwise perfect application. In short, it can hurt you more than it can help you. Don't be dumb.

## Harold Callahan, Dermatology

Start early and get advice from your residency director and a couple editors. Ask people in the department what they hate reading about. It is usually something that everyone writes about and becomes nauseating on the umpteenth time. Common mistakes are writing about exercise (especially long distance running) and comparing it to medicine or some sort of struggle.

*"It's like dating. Reveal your weirdness and insecurities early on and you can save a buttload of time not investing in places that are a poor match."*

*- Samuel Austin*

Honestly, stay away from struggle and any hardnock BS. No one cares how hard you had it going to public school from a working class family. You can play the working class angle, but don't look for pity. The people reading these are often older and have seen some shit (think about the 70's). Also, other applicants have come from third world countries, and their struggle will blow your struggle away. Parents being killed, warlords and famine kind of stuff. This principle holds true for diseases you might have. If it isn't a serious handicap then keep it to yourself.

Another theme, "TMI"(too much information) do not write about things that are too personal. Do not restate your CV!

Finally, most of all don't say that the moment that I knew I wanted to do radiology was when I looked at my grandmothers X-Ray..... or because I have acne or psoriasis I want to do Dermatology.

There are few musts. 1. state why you want to do that specific field and how you came to that conclusion 2. What do you plan to do in the field? Academia is the right answer, build on that.

The best advice is to try to explain that you are a normal person and give some background about yourself and how you came to where you are now, what motivates you and what you plan to do in the future.

I didn't tailor letters specifically to programs, but if you have a well written statement, this could be an easy sentence or two switch for each program that may make a difference. Not sure though.

## G. Michael Krauthamer, Emergency Medicine

It's hard to give advice on personal statements because they are, well, personal. That said, I was repeatedly advised the following: the personal statement is not a cover letter; don't reiterate your resume in your personal statement, and don't do anything too crazy or unintelligible e.g. poetry. I found the essay hard because the space is so limited, which makes the task of writing a coherent essay challenging. Make sure you have a trusted editor who can help you pair down your statement into a concise narrative.

Consider reading examples of "good" essays which you can find online, to get a sense of different ways to structure essays. Finally, start the essay early so you have time to edit it.

In the end I tried to link a few formative experiences that I had before and during medical school into a narrative about why I was passionate about medicine generally, and specifically how I arrived at choosing Emergency Medicine as a specialty. This helped me during interviews with questions such as, "why did you choose this specialty," to which I would respond, "I think I articulated this in my essay when I said…"

In so doing I was able to bring the interviewer's attention back to my essay, which I felt was strong. Often, in response to my citing my own essay in response to a question, a reviewer would say, "oh yeah, I liked when you wrote…" This provided an opening in which I was able to elaborate on areas I wanted to include in my essay but was unable to due to space restrictions, and to talk about topics I felt passionate about. The net effect was that my essay became a tool for engaging the interviewer in my responses.

## Burt Johnson, Urology

The personal statement was a challenge for me as I'm sure it was for every student, and will continue to be a challenge for students in the future. Getting started is the hardest part.

My strategy at the outset was first to put myself in the position of the reader. I imagined that I was a busy attending, and I was handed a stack of 20 or 30 applications. I had to take them home with me and do extra work in the evening to look them over. Despite enjoying this work, it also means take time away from reading to my kids or eating dinner with my wife or not getting to go play Thursday evening pickup hockey. Once I put myself in that position I knew that I had to make a personal statement short, professional, and yet engaging. Of course this is easier said than done.

*"The one thing that got me on track (and please don't judge me for this) was drinking three glasses of wine and just typing whatever came to mind. The next morning I woke up and read what I wrote down and was like wow, that was super honest."*

*-Alyssa Mendelson*

My personal constraint was that I was not allowed to write more than one page. The other element was each word in every sentence on the page had to be valuable. I simply thought, "what would I like to read about at the end of a long day in the OR, or a long clinic day when I'm sitting on my couch at 8 o'clock in the evening?"

My goal was to combine a captivating anecdote to catch the reader's attention, and then incorporate elements of my personality I wanted to emphasize throughout the rest of the personal statement. Before I started writing, I outlined the characteristics that I wanted to advertise and the talking points I wanted to elicit from an interviewer who may have read my personal statement. I then structured an anecdote or two (real, not fabricated) or talked about an experience that showed a particular characteristic about myself and how it applied to why I would make a good urologist.

I almost strategized this personal statement like a political speechwriter might organize talking points prior to delivering a speech or press junket. I just wanted to understand my audience and then deliver them a platter of words showing what I could bring to the table. It's a fine balance between professional writing and captivating writing. That being said, while I thought I employed an admirable strategy, I am not a particularly strong writer. Therefore it may have been a total flop, but I can tell you that while it may not have been in the 5% to 10% of essays or personal statements that get noticed and commented on interviews, it wasn't in the bottom five or 10% that excluded me from a lot of interviews. My personal statement was commented on by maybe four or five of the 13 programs that I interviewed at.

The other strategy that I did not employ, but would in hindsight, is to find a simple way to customize the personal statement to a geographic location. If there was a way to include one customized sentence in each personal statement and send them to individual programs, that may have taken me an additional 2 to 3 hours, but it may have yielded more interview offers. One possible way to stretch your geographic reach is through making a customized statement in your personal essay. This may be harder to do time efficiently if you're applying to a large number of programs.

However if there are at least 10 programs that you really want to interview at, it may be worth your time and effort. In hindsight, I wish I would have written my personal essay such that I could incorporate at least one or two lines where I could demonstrate specific interest in the program or surrounding geography.

## Calvin Barber, Anesthesia

I tried and tried to make my personal statement not be incredibly boring. I have talked to program directors, heads of departments, and interviewers about personal statements. Universally, they said that 90% personal statements are a complete waste of time, but the one time worth reading can be absolutely fascinating. Of course that's what we're all trying to do, be one of the 10% that writes a non-formulaic or captivating personal statement. I tried to write mine as an answer to the question that I thought everyone was going to ask. So if you can find that question then you have a place to start.

For me, it was obvious. I'm a very non-traditional, non-run-of-the-mill candidate, and the question that was clearly going to be on everyone's mind was:

"What are you doing here? Why here why did you make this choice?"

So that's what my personal statement was about. I think you can overthink the personal statement, but the best piece of advice I got regarding mine was when I was on my 15th revision and my advisor said to me, "You know… the enemy of good is… better."

Basically, it's done. Leave it alone, stop fiddling with it. And that's what I did. Lots of interviewers referred to it and they felt,

"Yeah, that was a question I was going to ask, and it's a very clear answer to it. So let's talk about something else."

That is what I wanted to do in every interview. I didn't want to rehash the same thing time after time after time.

I applied for anesthesia and also for combined pediatrics/anesthesia, and I didn't change my personal statement for each. Because I was applying for a combined program, I also had to apply to pediatrics on its own, and I did change my personal statement for that. There were some references to why I want to do anesthesia in my personal statement that I felt like I really need to change. For transitional programs, I did not change my statement.

It's very dangerous to step off the path into creative writing. Certainly, my first attempts at the personal statement were more like stories. They were too entertaining. They were too emotional, they were just too interesting, and I think it's distracting. For me, as I said earlier, focus on what they can ask, and talk about that. That was a useful way of grounding myself, at least in terms of a place to start.

> "Honestly, stay away from struggle and any hardnock BS … other applicants have come from third world countries, and their struggle will blow your struggle away. Parents being killed, warlords and famine kind of stuff. This principle holds true for diseases you might have. If it isn't a serious handicap then keep it to yourself."
>
> -Harold Callahan

I certainly did not personalize my statement for specific programs. I did try to hint at the geographic location because I'm in school in the East and my target for residency was the West. In interviews, I said I'm applying to programs only in the West - that's where I plan to be. I did not do that my personal statement.

## Whitney Alduron, Anesthesia

For my personal statement I wrote about the three things in life that matter most to me: my family, being active, and having a meaningful career. I received a lot of positive feedback about my statement during the interviews because it was relatively unique. My goal for the personal statement was to give programs a sense of who I am as a person and I think that came across very well. I did not customize any personal statements for geographic locations however I definitely realized that your personal statement can impact you either positively or negatively (geographically) depending on what you say. For example with regards to being active I talked about my passion for skiing and I think that was a benefit for programs in New England and out west but interestingly I did not receive any interview offers in the south or Midwest which I think may be directly related to my personal statement (although I can't be sure).

I think that if you are really trying to go somewhere specific it might be advantageous to write a customized personal statement talking about your connections to that area. Programs don't want to waste their time and resources interviewing candidates who have no interest in actually coming to the area.

## Tyler van Backer, General Surgery

Make it short and sweet. Program directors and evaluators have to read many statements. No one wants to read a million three-page essays. Aim for a page to two pages at maximum. I began thinking about the personal statement early and would just jot down random ideas that came to my mind in a word document. It made the whole brainstorming process a lot easier.

It seems kind of obvious, but the personal statement really needs to be something that comes from the heart. As some say, you can use the personal statement to address any shortcomings in your application (failed courses/boards), but make sure to spin them positively (i.e. what you learned, how you're preventing failures, things you're doing differently, etc.).

## Cameron Smith, Internal Medicine

The personal statement, depending on what field you are applying for, can be either a formality or weigh heavily on how you are perceived by a program. The advice I was given when writing my personal statement was to "stay within the lines" – not be too outlandish or extreme in any opinions, while at the same time effectively summarize what interests you about your particular field.

The personal statement should not be more than one page, typed, single-spaced, because longer personal statements often are an annoyance given programs receive hundreds to thousands of applications. You want to effectively demonstrate in that one page any experiences in your life, or personality traits that make you suited to be in the specific field to which you are applying.

> *"The net effect was that my essay became a tool for engaging the interviewer in my responses."*
>
> *- G. M. Krauthamer*

I was told that my personal statement was slightly unconventional. At the beginning of my PS, I included a small paragraph about a joke that I heard by a stand-up comedian at a comedy show years ago. Following that, I delved into what experience I had during med school, and in my personal life, that make me suited for internal medicine. I included one paragraph discussing my "scientific" side, and how the thought process involved in creating a differential diagnosis suited this side of me. I included another paragraph discussing my artistic nature, and how this field involved the art of patient interaction that I enjoyed. In the final paragraph, I addressed the anecdote that I opened with, and how it tied both the art and science of medicine together in a way that suited my future interests. The unconventionality came off as passionate and real, and at the same time it allowed for interesting discussion during my interview.

## Samuel Austin, Anesthesiology

I have a couple of advisors in my department who were essential to me not making an ass out of myself through the application process. The best advice I received about personal statements is that the content of 85% of them will be straight-down-the-middle and safe, but also unremarkable and therefore not very memorable. 10% will be memorable in a bad way and hurt the application. 5% will be memorable in a good way and help the application. I'm not a betting man (unless it's on Greyhounds and Powerball), so I took the safe route. I heard over and over again to write no more than one page, so write no more than one page.

Write about something you're passionate about. I drew parallels between one of my favorite pastimes, mountain biking, and anesthesiology. It served as a good conversation starter in several interviews and made it so I didn't have to write a painful, cheesy, "here's why I'm great" personal statement.

I didn't customize my statement for programs. I decided that I want to go to a place that was a great fit; if I wasn't putting my honest self out there then I would be doing myself and the program a disservice. It's like dating. Reveal your weirdness and insecurities early on and you can save a butt-load of time not investing in places that are a poor match.

# Making Deadlines? Submitting As Early As Possible?

## Mairin Jerome, PM & R

I submitted about 3 or 4 days late. My personal statement wasn't ready, so I delayed a couple of days. Ultimately, it worked out okay for me, but submitting right away would have been better. Every program does things differently, but it seems that many start reviewing the first round and send out interview invitations right away, whereas others wait until all applications are in and then review.

## Tyler van Backer, General Surgery

Completely my opinion, but applying early is important. It doesn't have to be at midnight when the application opens (and good luck getting into the website with the thousands of others), but have your application into programs with the first day. It doesn't have to be complete (and sometimes it's not possible since LORs can be submitted up until 10/1 and ERAS opens 9/15), but try to have everything complete on your end.

## Cameron Smith, Internal Medicine

The best advice for submitting the application is to do it on time. I would advise against waiting a day after the application is open to make minor changes to the personal statement. Submitting on time far supersedes any benefit these minor changes may have on your application. In my opinion, the application should be submitted on the first day.

## Harold Callahan, Dermatology

I don't think early submission is as important in dermatology as in other fields. Most programs do not start looking over applications until November. That being said they may look at them in order of submission, but I honestly doubt it is very important.

## Alyssa Mendelson, General Surgery

Submit your application on September 15. Some programs start sending interviews immediately. I got four interviews in the first two days. Don't miss the first wave!

## G. Michael Krauthamer, Emergency Medicine

There was a lot of prototypical medical student freneticism about posting residency applications to ERAS the minute this was allowed. I did not do this—I posted my application about a week after the ERAS system opened, and continued to apply to programs into early December. Apparently some programs will prefer really early applicants. I did not find this to be the case.

Suffice it to say, as long as you apply to programs in a relatively timely fashion (say within the first week or two after the system opens), you will probably be fine. That said, my esteemed colleagues in really competitive specialties (e.g. dermatology, radiology) insist that posting your application the day the system opens is paramount. I suspect that even in these specialties there is a tendency to exaggerate the importance of this. Common sense prevails here—you want to apply with enough time for programs to review your application and offer you a variety of dates for interviewing. The bulk of interviewing takes place in December and January, so obviously, applying earlier is better.

# Letters of Recommendation

## Calvin Barber, Anesthesia

I felt my letters of recommendation were a significant strength of my application. There were several places where people commented on how strong those letters were and I think that was a big deal. In that context, I think one of the key things for my letters was the fact that I have been hanging out with the anesthesiologists for about a year prior to my application as I tried to figure out whether or not anesthesia was appealing to me.

During my third year, through a chance conversation, I got interested in anesthesia as a possibility, and started going to Grand Rounds. I never particularly mingled with the anesthesiologists early on, but was just there and people noticed and gradually started to invite me to other things like journal clubs. I spent a couple days shadowing so that I was a presence, and I was known by the department. So when I decided that anesthesia was what I was going to do, it was pretty easy to find people that thought they knew me personally - knew me well enough that they could write a letter of recommendation that was not just a form letter. One that was about me specifically - and I think that shows in the letters that get written.

My letters, for what it's worth, were written by the chief of anesthesiology at my home institution, the anesthesia program director at my school, plus one NICU attending from a rotation I did fairly early my fourth year, and a pediatrician who lectured in the first and second year medical school and also was one of the attendings during my pediatric clerkship - so someone that I felt knew me in different contexts and over a long period of time. Those were my four letters of recommendation.

## G. Michael Krauthamer, Emergency Medicine

For me, letters emphasized in particular my professionalism. During interviews, programs explicitly stated that they were impressed with my letters of recommendation, which I think indicates that above all, programs want to make sure they are hiring committed, professional residents. The take home point is, that as one approaches the clinical years, perhaps more importantly than out-gunning your colleagues, or honoring all of your rotations, is conveying a sense of professionalism and maturity; even if you don't ace your shelf exams you will demonstrate your value as a part of the team, and your colleagues and mentors will be more than happy to support you when it comes time to apply for residency.

# Burt Johnson, Urology

As for individual sections on the ERAS, such as research, work, and volunteer sections, my philosophy was to be very conservative about how I portray all of my experiences. I never wanted to exaggerate any accomplishments or experiences because I wanted to be very comfortable when it came time to interview in person just being honest. I didn't want to be interviewed under false pretenses. There is actually some literature on PubMed about how many applicants actually put inaccurate or exaggerated information on their applications, particularly in research sections. I think it's too much of a risk to overstate what you have done or mistakenly say you published something that wasn't actually published. I personally didn't want to put too many things on my ERAS because I felt I would come off as unfocused and a bit scatterbrained. I looked at ERAS as a way to portray myself in the best possible way and rather than listing off a large quantity, I wanted to present a focused approach where many of the experiences could be connected together to tell my story.

# 10

# THE INTERVIEW TRAIL

*Program Selection, Logistics, and*

*Pre/Post-Interview Socials*

# Program Selection

## Calvin Barber, Anesthesia

I very specifically targeted a West Coast residency, and I came from an east coast school. I'm also a fairly unusual candidate shall we say; I'm the oldest student in my graduating class and have been successful in a prior public industry before returning to medical school.

I applied to a fairly broad spectrum of places because California has a lot of anesthesia programs, and Oregon, Washington, Utah and Colorado all were within my area of interest, the West essentially. I was surprised by some of the places that I didn't get interviews because they were my backup programs in my mind. It is certainly possible that they register that or have an algorithm that they use to figure out whether someone will actually come to their program or whether they will be wasting an interview. I cannot answer that because they did not interview me, and I did not have the chance to get that sense from him. Certainly there were programs where thought I could get interviews, but in hindsight it feels to me that if I had done an away rotation there, I would have been interviewed.

For me, program selection was all about geography. I was very specific about where I was applying, basically nothing east of Colorado. Ultimately, I think geography probably is the biggest thing if you have a completely free choice. If you're specialty is really difficult to get into than you just go wherever you get an invitation.

If you think you're a strong candidate, you get to choose, why would you pick anything other geography? I guess some people are really excited by particular names, but that just isn't a big deal for me. It was much more about, is it going to be -20° at any time while I'm there? Is the sun going to shine, will the sky be blue? Will the ocean lap against the beach?

> *"If you think you're a strong candidate, you get to choose. Why would you pick anything other than geography?"*
>
> *- Calvin Barber*

Additionally, I spoke to my advisors and anesthesia, a lot. I made contact with alumni that were at programs outside my home program. I made contact with them pretty early on because I was deciding where to do away rotations.

I applied to 16 anesthesia programs and I got 8 interviews. I applied to two combined programs (peds/anesthesia), I got one interview there, and I applied to probably about six or so transitional year programs and got three interviews. About 50% was my interview acquisition rate.

With respect to responding to interview invitations, I had backup. There were times when I had gotten a message from the program and I would forward the message to my wife who had my password and access to my account. She would login and see what it was, and we would try to communicate by text and then she would email the programs. Different programs did things differently for sure, some contacted only through the ERAS system and some communicated directly with me by email, it was very variable. Generally that whole thing was pretty smooth. I had a couple of programs who contacted me to say that I was essentially on the reserve list and didn't have an interview slot, but they were keeping my details on file. I think those were probably real, as opposed to just a form letter saying were keeping you on file. The reason I think that is because they were programs that my advisor had personal connections with. So I think the letters were genuine responses to not having offered me an interview in the first skim through. After they had been contacted and asked to take a serious look at the application, they still didn't have interview slots in both those programs. Ultimately I didn't interview at either of those programs, but they did stay in contact.

There are a couple programs I wish had interviewed at, but I don't think I'd gone there anyway. I think if I hadn't done an away rotation, I think I wouldn't have gotten an interview and I would be answering this very differently. But basically I come back to what I said in a previous conversation, the magic number is one. You find a program that you really like and they really like you, after that nothing else matters. Everyone freaks out, and it drives some so crazy with the idea that all I have to have is 12 interviews in order to have a 95% chance of matching. It's nonsense, all that crap is complete nonsense.

## G. Michael Krauthamer, Emergency Medicine

The general rule of thumb is that the more competitive the specialty, the more programs you should apply to. For emergency medicine, (assuming competitive step scores, passing grades in the preclinical years, strong letters of recommendations and honors in sub-internships), if a student interviews at 10 programs, the likelihood of matching is quoted as being above 90%. I applied to 30 programs and was invited to interviews at 15 of these, which seemed about average.

## Burt Johnson, Urology

The way I selected programs was primarily based on geography selected by me and my lovely girlfriend. Together, we simply went down the list of all the programs and basically said yes or no to living there. Based on preliminary geographic qualification or disqualification, I selected programs based on what I had heard about them from my advisors, other students who had applied to urology, and name recognition (for worse or better).

If I'm being perfectly honest, there is an insufficient amount of information on program websites and on forums to guide you in selecting programs that would be a good fit for you. I think this is a primary reason why the average number of applications submitted each year is growing in Urology. There is very little way for applicants to distinguish programs other than name recognition and geography prior to visiting programs on interview day. In fact most program websites are not updated frequently and have numerous errors on them.

There is no metric for quality of life during residency that programs can objectively demonstrate to you. And while it's taboo to want quality of life over the best possible training situation, the reality is that most residents care about quality of life.

I applied to 39 programs, and received 14 interview offers plus I didn't have to interview at one of my away rotations. Because of scheduling conflicts I had to cancel two of my interviews. It is important to have some method for checking your email or checking your ERAS frequently to ensure you respond to interview offers as soon as possible. No matter how obnoxious, your phone needs to push your email constantly to you for that two-month period of time or however long it is, and you need to be in a place where you can constantly check ERAS if you need to.

The sad reality can be that if you don't respond to an interview request within the first 15 minutes, you are not going to get your first choice interview date, and this can cause you to cancel interviews because of conflicts (I learned the hard way). If I was smarter, more hard-working, and diligent, I would have made a calendar of all the programs that I applied to and what days they typically interview. This way I could quickly reference it when an offer came my way and choose dates that had the least probability of being in conflict with other programs.

In fact one of the programs Jefferson sent out an email via you ERAS saying that they invited 50 people for an interview, but that they only have room to interview 40, and thus it would be first reply first serve. This is a bizarre strategy and one that I don't necessarily agree with, but when you have the luxury of having 350 applicants for three positions, you can do whatever you want.

## Samuel Austin, Anesthesiology

My criteria were mixed. I wanted to train at the "best" place I could in order to open doors and allow for as many options as possible down the road (commitment makes me queasy). "Best" translated to the biggest name place early on. Therefore, I applied to the 10-12 biggest names in U.S. hospitals. I also applied to places in cool cities that I felt would offer a good life outside of work. I have never lived outside of New England and set my sights west, as residency is a finite period of time to go live somewhere else.

I was actually surprised by many of the larger institutions. I felt that at some places the faculty and residents seemed completely burnt out and unhappy, running in a rat race to garner the most publications or pick up extra shifts to send their kids to the best private schools, which they of course wanted everyone to know about. I had never been to an Ivy-League anything before and was nervous about visiting some of the places I was fortunate to be invited to. In the end, it was surprising how normal the residents, staff, and faculty seemed at most these places. Again, good people are everywhere.

My advisors were extremely helpful. They helped me create the list of places to apply based on the characteristics of programs that I valued ("door opener programs", larger academic centers, high-stakes and high-acuity cases, centralized rather than decentralized (i.e., fewer rather than multiple training sites), strength in critical care, geography, personality of the department, type of research taking place there, and so on…). From my advisors I gleaned many inside tips that weren't available on the internet, especially relating to the "feel" of each department compared to my home department which I'd grown to love.

I sent 20 applications out and got interviews from 17 of them. There were programs who surprised me by inviting me to interview and others who surprised me when they didn't invite me. I emailed a couple of preliminary programs to inform them of my interest sometime in January, which was likely too late, but didn't hear from them anyhow. Some of my friends contacted programs they had interest in and were granted an interview. It can't hurt to try.

## Alyssa Mendelson, General Surgery

This was a nightmare. At the time, I had no idea if I wanted to stay local or leave and go live on the other side of the country. I didn't know if I wanted to be in a big city or a rural environment. I honestly was like, "all I know is UVM, how am I supposed to know what other programs to apply to?" I guess this is where away rotations could have helped me, but I still would have only done one or two.

I ended up casting a really wide net, and then as I did my first few interviews I found out a lot about what aspects of a program I really liked. I was able to narrow down interviews I accepted after that. This method is certainly more expensive, and in hindsight I really wish I'd given geography more consideration. When I got off the plane in Rochester, MN, I seriously was like what the bleep am I doing here? A great program in a location you hate isn't going to work out. Make sure you really think about where you do and don't want to live.

Also, during my interviews, a ton of residents gave me the advice "Stick close to family and friends. Residency is hard enough on its own, having support somewhere nearby is key." When it came to making my rank list, this advice certainly stuck with me. Most academic surgery programs are 5-7 years long – that's a long time to live in a place you hate and without family or close friends.

I ended up applying to 44 programs and got interviews at I think at approximately 34-35 of these programs. Obviously I applied to far too many – this was my "wide-net" method. My recommendation is to schedule all of the interviews you can, and then start to pick and choose as you see who is interested in you and who isn't. Also, a lot of times I would get invitations for programs in the same city at different times, so I wouldn't be able to schedule those two interviews close together initially. It is perfectly ok to email a program coordinator and request to be placed on a wait list for another day if it's more convenient for your travel schedule. This process is expensive, and if you can visit two programs in one trip, definitely try to do it.

Of the 34 interview invitations I received, I did 13. I had 14 scheduled, but I had to cancel an interview at one of the best surgical programs in the country because I got the flu. Note: Get the flu shot, wash your hands, and don't sit near people on a plane wearing a mask that is only covering their mouth and not their nose.

## Harold Callahan, Dermatology

In dermatology, you apply to all the programs. Unfortunately, it has become the name of the game. Sent out 115 applications, received 9 interview offers.

Early bird gets the worm these days. Set your phone up with a VIP ringtone and vibration for eras messages. Be sure to have a program on your mobile device that allows you to open eras. Safari does not work on iphones. Instead I used UC Browser. There are a number of programs that you can use.

Realistically any interview that involved flying cost me around $600. I would still have gone on more. Be sure to sign up for TSA pre clearance. This is a life saver. I only stayed with trustworthy friends and hotels only. Too much to risk.

## Whitney Alduron, Anesthesia

Choosing which programs to apply to was by far the most fun part of the entire application process. I remember sitting down with my advisor and saying, "I want to apply to every program that is within a 2 hour drive of skiing" and that was my criteria.

I also ended up applying to some big-name programs that were not as close to skiing just for the hell of it. I am originally from Connecticut and have lived my entire life in New England. That was both a blessing and a curse because I really had no geographical or family connections to any programs outside of New England, and it was significantly more difficult to obtain interviews in those areas. However I did interview at every single program I applied to in New England except one.

For anesthesia, it's extremely difficult and inconsistent to get national rankings on programs. It seems as though most program directors have a sense of which programs have a good/great reputation and which ones less so. My advisor is the program director at my home institution, and his input was invaluable when it came to deciding which programs to apply to and which I would be competitive at (since there is no official ranking system).

At the end of the day it seemed to me that there were a handful of excellent programs, the vast majority were very good and there were only a few bad programs. Being from New England, name recognition (I hate to admit it) was important to me, however I did not necessarily feel that correlated with quality. Often it did not correlate with the program director's opinion of the program. For example, in New England there are three Ivy League program, but only one of the anesthesia residency programs associated with these colleges is a top-tier program. When my dad said to me "why don't you want to go to the anesthesia program associated with Ivy League __?" and I told him "Because it's not as good as the program associated with State University ___" he was shocked.

Honestly when it truly came down to deciding my rank list I ended up choosing the location I wanted to live over everything else because I knew I would get a very good education at every single place I interviewed. I remember at one interview in Boston, the program director told me he could not honestly tell me I would get a better education at his program than at another top 10 program, and therefore it was up to me to decide if this was a place I wanted to train and live.

Anesthesia has both advanced and categorical spots so I applied to 26 anesthesia programs and 10 preliminary medicine programs. I did not apply to any transitional year programs. I attended all eight anesthesia interviews that I was offered.

I was offered one preliminary medicine interview that I did not attend. At the end of the interview season my statistics were broken into thirds: I was offered about one third interviews (8/26), I received a rejection letter from one third of the programs (9/26) and I did not hear at all from one third of the programs (9/26).

I was honestly very shocked that I did not receive more interview offers and I was disappointed that I did not hear at all from one third of the programs. It is bullshit that you spend all this time, energy, and money on your application to not even have them respond with a "thanks but no thanks" and leave you hanging for the duration of the interview season. It also puts you in an awkward position with regards to emailing and asking for an interview because you are never sure whether you are doing it too early or too late if you haven't heard anything. I would've rather received a rejection email than hear nothing.

To me, the interview process seemed very similar to medical school in the sense that it was very arbitrary. I received three interviews at top 10 programs however I did not get interviews at some less competitive programs and truly believe it was due to geography. I received all but one interview in New England, two interviews out west (near ski areas), but no interview offers in California, the Midwest or the South.

On my away rotation I met students from other schools with similar backgrounds to mine (grades, board scores, etc. ), and they were really great, awesome, normal people. Obviously we got to comparing where we had gotten interviews and although there was some overlap the majority of decisions seemed arbitrary as to who they invited. For example, we all applied to the same 3 schools in the Pacific Northwest and none of us ended up getting the same interview.

I never had a situation where I was offered an interview, but did not get a date because I did not respond soon enough. That being said I didn't always end up with my first choice date either. I honestly feel I was very lucky because I like my home program very much. I didn't feel the need to go on significantly more interviews because I felt if I would rather stay at my home program over the other program, then I wouldn't bother emailing and requesting an interview or freaking out that I did not get one. For me, eight was plenty of interviews.

## Tyler van Backer, General Surgery

Geography was important for me. My fiancée and I only wanted to be in the northeast, which cut out a lot of programs. I also am not a fan of NYC, so that cut out a lot programs. For the most part, the better known names were better programs, but there certainly are some programs that don't get shown on the TV dramas, yet are still top-tier and extremely competitive programs.

My advisor was really helpful in terms of making my rank list and contacting programs on my behalf. I also spoke with our Chair of Surgery. If someone knows you well, talk with them. I solicited feedback about programs and malignancy issues from interns and friends who had gone into surgery the year before me, which was helpful because they had a more recent feel for programs. I used a website that isn't up any longer from the American Board of Surgery, which is really unfortunate because it was helpful. I also used AMA's FREIDA for information.

When I looked at programs websites, I took it with a grain of salt since any program can look spectacular on paper. Depending what is important to you, try to seek that information out from current residents. To do this, I searched the 'current residents' tab, if they were available, and looked for my school. Usually alumni are willing to give you an honest appraisal of a program.

I sent out 24 applications, initially, then had a moment of panic and sent out an additional two a couple days later. I was offered 16 interviews and accepted 14. I think 14 interviews was more than enough. I'm glad that I went on those, though, because there were a fair amount of programs I really would not be happy at, despite my best efforts to vet the program ahead of time.

Before getting any interviews, I tried to list all of the dates for each program that I applied to in an Excel spreadsheet and noted the ones that overlapped with other programs. This was only possible for those that listed their dates on their website (~2/3 for my selections). For those that didn't, I listed the information they gave, if any and put the document in my Dropbox so that when I got an invite, I was able to check the dates and try to pick one that didn't overlap with another possible/confirmed interview.

This process is expensive, but it's obviously very important- it's not a time to try to be cheap.

I had an iPhone and Safari doesn't work with ERAS. Instead, use Mercury Web Browser and set your homepage to the ERAS login page. In order to view the page, you have to change the settings of how the browser displays what type it is to Firefox or IE. It's in the settings tab at the bottom of the app. The first time you login, it will ask if you want to save your ID/password for the autofill feature, which I found helpful for quickness of logging into the system.

It is vitally important to respond ASAP. Perfect example: I left my phone on as long as I could before a less than 90 minute flight to Philly for Step 2. My phone was off for about an hour fifteen minutes and a couple minutes after I turned it off, I received an invite. When I turned it back on about an hour later, two of the four dates had been filled. Several of my friends have relayed similar stories. In order to know when you get an interview invite, there are two main services that you should add to your "VIP alerts" (by making a contact card for each). The three emails I put in were "noReply@aamc.org", "noreply@eraspod.aamc.org", and "interviews@interviewbroker.com".

To do this, I made a contact with the emails and then went into my mail app and set those emails to be VIP. I also had my email automatically push to my phone (important so you get the email as soon as it comes). Under settings >> notifications >> mail >> VIP, you can adjust the sounds that a VIP email will make a different (hopefully noticeable) sound from your regular email sound. Be wary, though, I also did receive a personalized email from a program, directly, so remaining glued to your phone is still important, as well. Along those lines, try to not be in the OR or on a rotation where you can't look at your phone every so often during September, October, November, and early December. Usually, my invites came during October and November, but I did receive a couple in September and in December, as well.

## Cameron Smith, Internal Medicine

Geography was high on my list when considering places to be for residency. I had reasons to be closer to family in Los Angeles, and so about 50% of the programs I applied to were in California. At the same time, I didn't want to limit myself and kept an open mind, so I applied fairly broadly to major cities like Boston, Chicago, and New York. I would definitely recommend sitting down with your specialty advisor or residency director at your home institution to discuss programs.

Most of the information I got about programs was through word of mouth. I ended up sending out about 35 total applications for internal medicine. I was offered 17 interviews and attended 14. In retrospect, 35 may have been a few too many, but at the same time I erred on the side of applying to programs I was ambivalent about, in case I would find out information throughout the process that may be positive about that particular program. I would definitely recommend setting up push email for those who have smart phones, to be able to respond as quickly as possible for interview offers. Spots can fill up very quickly, especially for programs that use online calendar sites where people can select a date they are interested in.

# Mairin Jerome, PM & R

I did not really have a specific advisor from my school in PM & R to help me weed through programs, so I mainly went with geography and name recognition. There are about 5 PM & R programs that are considered "the best" in the field, so I chose those and then went with geography and general reputation of institutions.

I ultimately applied to too many programs and wish I had connected with someone from my field who was familiar with programs to help narrow. After I submitted my application, the doximity review of residency programs came out with ranking of programs within fields. I relied on that to add a couple more applications, and then ultimately learned that this is a popularity poll.

Program websites were frequently not up to date and had different program directors listed, outdated rotation and call schedules etc., so take the info from a website with a grain of salt.

I applied to about 50 PM & R programs which was too many. I ultimately received 18 PM & R interview offers and attended 12 of them. I had to choose between several programs because interview dates conflicted.

Prelim year was more difficult. I was not organized about this and sent both my prelim medicine and TY applications out very late (probably at least 10-14 days). I applied to about 35 medicine programs and 15 TY programs, all roughly based on where I was applying geographically for PM & R. I ended up with 3 prelim medicine interviews and 2 transitional year interviews. This is a pretty low rate of return, but apparently is not that unusual. Many people applying in competitive specialties also apply for a prelim year as a backup. I even met an EM applicant on a TY interview.

Some PM & R programs offer a first year as a categorical position or have a deal with a TY year at their institution so that if you match there for PM & R, you automatically match for their TY year.

If you have a home program, double check that they take prelims. I mistakenly thought my home hospital did, but found out after the fact that the prelim positions they have are reserved for candidates going into advanced residencies at my hospital (anesthesia or radiology), and did not accept people applying for my field (hence my late and frantic flurry of additional prelim applications).

# Logistics: Costs, Travel, & Lodging

## Whitney Alduron, Anesthesia

I feel like one of the lucky ones with regards to how easy the interview season was. With the exception of two interviews out west, all were in New England and I drove to all of them. In Connecticut, I stayed with my family and in Massachusetts I stayed with friends and at a hotel. My favorite part of the interview season was finally feeling as though I was being treated as a professional. About half of the places I interviewed offered me a free hotel stay and for the first time I finally felt like all of the hard work I've put in over the past 3 1/2 years was beginning to pay off.

Residency interviews make you feel like a valued individual and (although there are still periods of groveling for interviews that you want or writing emails showing your desire to be ranked highly) for the most part you have the upper hand. Out west I was doing my away rotation when I was interviewed so I did not have to travel, and I flew to one interview on the West Coast from Utah which was obviously significantly easier than flying from the East Coast. I think in total I spent between $800 and $1000 for the entire interview season.

## Mairin Jerome, PM & R

I ended up spending about $7000. This was relatively unavoidable with last minute invitations that required last minute plane reservations.

I applied for a travel rewards credit card ahead of time, which was helpful and at least I was able to redeem points on some of my travel expenses. Ultimately, I went to 17 interviews (one of which was late and done via Skype) and went to two informational sessions. I would not travel a far distance just for an info session, but I was going to be in the area anyway for interviews. If you are going to be in an area anyway, it is worth calling a program to see if they can fit you in around the same time (I was able to do this with one preliminary interview).

I had difficulty scheduling my PM & R interviews in the same areas of the country in a convenient way because the interview season was so long, dates were relatively inflexible, and the offers came in over the course of 2 months.

I am happy with the number of interviews I went on. I went on 12 for my PM & R rotations, and ranked 10-11 of those programs. I attended all interviews I was offered for my intern year and 2 informational sessions (one for a TY year and one for a prelim med year that was connected to a PM & R program). I am glad I went to the info session days. One of them was terrible and I may have otherwise ranked it if I had not gone.

I stayed with friends wherever possible - though if your friends are noisy and the sleeping arrangements are not great, I would recommend paying for a hotel if it's before an important interview. A couple of my programs paid for the hotels, which was great. For the really important ones, I traveled an extra day ahead of time just in case of travel delays in the winter. Getting out to your interview city in advance also gives you an opportunity to experience the city and environment.

> *"For the really important ones, I traveled an extra day ahead of time just in case of travel delays in the winter."*
>
> *- Mairin Jerome*

Many programs advertise discounted rates with local hotels, but I didn't find the deals to be deals at all, so I used the "name your own price" feature on Priceline a lot. Same applies to car rentals if I needed one. Keep in mind that in some places, parking is an extra charge at most hotels in a city.

## Burt Johnson, Urology

I spent in the neighborhood of $3000 total on interviews. I went on 12 interviews, two thirds of those were drivable, but required a night stay in a hotel - say average of $100 on a per interview basis - maybe $250 all costs/interview.

In hindsight, I felt like I got the perfect amount of interviews. I applied to 39 programs, got 14 interview offers, and one program that would rank me for the away month I did. I ended up going on 12 interviews due to scheduling/travel conflicts. I wasn't particularly concerned that I wouldn't match, but it was always in the back of my mind. If I had eight or fewer, I would've been a little bit more nervous.

I stayed almost exclusively in hotels. I thought that it was worth the investment and interviews were too important to save $50-$80 x 12, considering the amount of debt each of us carries. The risk is obvious, you may not get a good night of sleep, you may be disrupted, and it's just too risky. At two or three interviews, I stayed with friends who understood my position and knew I had a professional interview, so they were very accommodating. I typically also stayed extra time at those places so that I could spend time with my friends and not feel like I had to stay up late one night drinking beers when I had an interview the next day.

I never rented a car. The programs that weren't near airports that I interviewed were all within driving distance. Programs to which I flew, I took public transportation or Uber or taxis etc. Some cars can be rented for as little as $11 a day which I found to be quite amazing. If I could rent a car for $11 a day consistently I probably would not own a car. Many of the applicants I talked to were able to get great deals like this for rental cars on Priceline. When renting, consider the time it will take to pick up and drop off a car (unless I think if you use National) and parking. There will be times where you will be rushed to get to the airport after your interview, either to your next interview or to get home, just take that into account.

Last item, I had an interview in San Francisco in mid-December so I booked my flight for a day early. They had one of their worst rain storms in 10 years which basically shut down all incoming flights after mine. Considering planning for storms if you have the luxury.

## Tyler van Backer, General Surgery

I spent probably around $3,000, which was with staying with friends and keeping a very tight geographic location. A more realistic amount if you don't fly and stay in nice(r) hotels (I learned my lesson staying at the cheapest hotel I could find on priceline…) is around $4,000 or $5,000. With that in mind, using the "name your own price" part of Priceline can be a good tool if you know the area hotels and can compare the map to a google map and look at the reviews of hotels in that area. I'm glad that I went on the number that I did. I found there were a couple of programs that I thought I would like and turned out to be disappointing.

I stayed with family/friends for three interviews. It was nice to save money, but, at the same time, it sometimes was harder because I didn't have my own space. It was great to see everyone, but I definitely felt like I stayed up later than I wanted to socialize, which was hard. Not the end of the world, though, and nice to have a better bed than a hotel.

## Alyssa Mendelson, General Surgery

I'd say I spent somewhere in the neighborhood of $5000-6000. I traveled all over the country, and plane tickets were really expensive. I also didn't have too many "connections" in the areas that I interviewed at, so I almost always had to stay in a hotel.

Hotel tip: Use the Priceline "name your own price" thing. If you select the area around your program, you can get really nice hotels (4-star +) for really cheap. I used this in 3 large cities and had a great experience with it.

## Samuel Austin, Anesthesiology

I spent around $5,000 in total. My school makes us meet with a financial advisor early on during the first year of medical school. I was advised to set aside a little bit of money each month or with each loan disbursement to prepare for residency travel, which I did. It allowed me to not have to take out additional loans and I was able to not worry about finances when traveling. That said, take out the money if you have to. I'd err on the side of visiting too many places than too few. You're probably in way over your head by the time you're reading this book, anyhow. It's only money…

I stayed with friends and at hotels. It is already stressful enough being on the road and interviewing several times a week, so I prioritized places to stay that had small fitness centers so I could exercise and decompress (i.e., to get my swell on). Often there will be a discounted rate for medical centers at area hotels. You can ask if you didn't receive explicit information about this from the program coordinator.

## Cameron Smith, Internal Medicine

I was lucky to not spend much by taking advantage of staying with friends/family members who lived close to programs. I also had fewer flights than others to pay for because most of the programs I applied to were in California, and I was able to drive to most places.

# Pre / Post Interview Dinners

## Calvin Barber, Anesthesia

My big thing, not just in interviews, but residents dinner the night before and on away rotations, frankly everything in life, my big thing is don't be fake. All these things that you hear, about things you must do and mustn't do…

"you must never drink alcohol at the resident's dinner…"

To me, if you don't drink alcohol at the resident's dinner, I won't trust you because I'd be concerned that you are afraid that something that is inside you is going to come out and be revealed. What are you so afraid for? Who are you? What is it that you're hiding?… that troubles me. If you never drink alcohol then fine, don't have a beer. If you do drink alcohol, then drink at the resident's dinner. Don't pretend to be somebody you're not. I may see the world that way because I'm European, but there you go.

Why pretend to be somebody that you're not? The whole point of the match process is figuring out where you fit. If you pretend to be somebody you're not and you match there, you've got to carry on pretending to be that person. That makes no sense to me at all. I know some people are vociferous, but do not drink at the residency parties. My question is - who are you? You're trying to hide from everybody. I would flat out not allow someone who did that into my program.

> *"If you know you can hang with the big boys then go for it. If not, stick to juice."*
>
> *– Harold Callahan (on drinking at socials)*

If you can go to residency dinners, I think it's good. Do not expect to get great information. Everyone's on their best behavior, you can't tell who they've made come to the dinner and who they told 'please don't come to dinner.' I did not find them to be tremendously illuminating - the residents said the same thing at every program I went to. They all seem to like each other and love the program, life was good. And again it's a red flag thing. You go to all the residency dinners, you may find one's just a nightmare. Actually having said that, I went to one residency dinner which was in a bar, and we were served water. This immediately says this is not a program you want to be a part of.

## Alyssa Mendelson, General Surgery

I never had more than two drinks. You are being judged on your professionalism, just be smart. I only remember one person who had too much to drink, and honestly it was just embarrassing to watch. They were interrupting the residents who were talking with us, stumbled back to the bar to get another drink, etc.

I never had residents try to influence me to "party" with them, so I can't comment on that. All I'm going to say is that you have an interview bright and early in the morning…do you want to be the person who falls asleep during the "program overview" presentation?

I only missed two pre-interview receptions and both were due to travel disasters. People always asked if you went or had a good time, but no one seemed to mind that my travel interfered with the reception. The interview day is certainly far more important than the reception.

## Samuel Austin, Anesthesia

I don't drink much, but I did have a glass of wine or a beer at most dinners out of social convention more than anything. Be slick. Don't overindulge and make yourself stand out for the wrong reasons. Have you ever seen James Bond get wasted? No? Then you probably shouldn't get hammered. If the residents are getting saucy, it's probably a bad idea to follow their lead. They already have the spot; you don't.

Go to the dinner if you can! It's a great way to get a decent meal when you probably haven't had one in a long time, and, most importantly, to do so for free. Just be friendly and conversational. There's no secret to it. I learned more about the program from observing the residents at these dinners than I did from the interview day. Further, nearly every program asked if I had gone to the dinner the night prior. Most of these places asked who I met, so try to remember 2-3 of the residents you met the night before. Remember, every dinner was "great" and everybody you met seemed "wonderful". No exceptions.

## G. Michael Krauthamer, Emergency Medicine

Many programs will offer you opportunities to socialize with residents before, during and after interviews. These are great opportunities to talk to residents about nitty-gritty details such as pay, schedule, and resident happiness. They will not think you a lazy greedy slob for asking how much a resident gets paid, or how vacations are organized.

Most programs offer pre-interview resident socials, generally there is alcohol at these functions, and sometimes it will be free. Be careful not to overdo it; the last person you want to be when meeting your potential new colleagues is be the sloppy drunk. Similarly if you are socially awkward in large groups, feel free to skip pre-interview socials; simply make up a polite excuse for not attending, it's not expected and you don't want to undermine your confidence the night before the interview by feeling like the weirdo in the corner who doesn't know how to make friends; you will have ample opportunity to talk to residents during your interview day.

## Harold Callahan, Dermatology

Be personable and have a good time. Do not be negative and don't be too talkative. This is probably the hardest to advise. You can teach social skills in a paragraph. With regards to drinking: if you know you can hang with the big boys, then go for it. If not, stick to juice.

## Whitney Alduron, Anesthesiology

I attended all of the interview dinners and I think they are a great way to see if you would fit in with the current residents. One thing I noticed that I needed to watch out for was that I began basing the program off of the other applicants. I started thinking "will these people be friends of mine?" and obviously that's not the right thing to do because you never know whether the program is at the top of their list or not. If you judge a program based on who else is interviewing there then you're not getting a true sense of the program. I remember one interview dinner I went to and about half of the applicants were on their cell phones texting or on Facebook/Instagram/Snapchat and I just thought it was so rude, and I thought to myself that I would never want to come to a place with people like this. Later, I had to remember these individuals were not actually representative of the program.

> *"I went to one residency dinner which was in a bar, and we were served water which immediately says this is not a program you want to be a part of."*
>
> *- Calvin Barber*

## Burt Johnson, Urology

What I can tell you from my personal experience on the urology interview trail is that most urology residents, attendings, and applicants are laid-back folks. Read the room, but certainly having a couple drinks is appropriate. At every interview, we had beers or drinks and some food, and it was very low-key. If you don't drink then don't drink, but if you normally drink, then being at a residency interview dinner shouldn't stop you from doing so. The people that you will be working with also like to have a good time, and there is no reason to hide that. No need to be the person that drinks eight beers when everyone else is having one or two with dinner. That's just being silly and careless.

Aside from the drinking discussion, residency interview socials are somewhat helpful. I felt that it was a good way to get to know the residents and get a good feel of the atmosphere and culture of the program. Know the programs are on their best behavior and can ask particular residents not to go. Thus you may get a slightly skewed perception, just keep it in mind.

One program had a pre-interview social at an upscale lounge bar, and fortuitously there also happened to be a fashion show that night. Another takeaway from a social is how much the program or the program director cares about the residents having a good time. The interview social isn't just about the applicants but also a time for the residents to have a little fun themselves. Often on the interview day, the program basically shut down and there were almost no surgeries on that day. This means a day off for the residents and they can have fun the night before and I think they enjoy it. Do think consciously of the group of residents that gets completely hammered on the interview social, it may indicate an outlet for a very stressful program.

Talking to fellow applicants who had done away rotations at other programs was incredibly helpful. You do have to put some faith in what other people are saying about programs, but the alternative is getting information only from interview day. On interview day, it's difficult to assess things like quality-of-life, culture, and general atmosphere. Everyone will say at every program that they're all friends, and they all work really well together, and all the attendings are lovely, and that no one ever throws instruments, or verbally abuses anyone, and every hospital gets a great surgical experience with surgical independence, and call isn't that bad and yada yada yada.

A few programs will recognize their limitations or their weaknesses, and you should not see this as a sign of inferiority, but rather a sign of honesty and respect to the applicants. While you do have to be careful listening to folks who have done an away month, and you certainly should take their comments with a grain of salt, if impressions by one person are validated by many others, I think it's safe to say that they're not making it up.

In general, while on the urology interview trail, I never thought that anyone was making anything up to deceive me. It just felt like a fairly frank conversation with most people, especially towards the tail end of interview season. At the beginning, fellow applicants were hesitant with what they should say, what they shouldn't say, and who might talk about things etc. By the end of interview season, applicants stopped giving a shit and were willing to be honest with you after they saw you at five other interview days.

Everyone roughly interviews at the same places, but everybody likes something different so they stop caring if you know about programs. The part where it becomes difficult to assess another applicant's comments about a place they did in a way rotation, is that you don't quite know what that person's personality is like or what they consider difficult working conditions or what they think is a good quality-of-life. Everybody has a different perception and baseline for those particular features.

## Jennifer Tango, Emergency Medicine

I would say just don't drink too much! You should know your limits and stop much before you hit that. I think it is fine to have a drink or two to help settle the nerves and facilitate conversation with people you've never met. Just don't overdo it. That strategy seemed to work fine for me at this interview because before rank lists were due the program director wrote me an email with specific details of things that we had discussed on my interview, saying how he would be happy if I matched at his program. I think my 2 beers that night had been perfectly titrated to effect.

## Cameron Smith, Internal Medicine

Don't be afraid to have one or two drinks at your dinners. Feel it out. If it seems like you would be the only person having a drink, I would advise against ordering one. If you do drink, and everyone is having drinks, don't feel shy about having one. It goes without saying that you probably should not be drinking too much during these dinners.

I attended about 50% of the dinners at places I interviewed. I would advise going to these dinners, because it can give you a chance to get to know the residents better, and discuss the program in a less formal environment. However, don't feel like it is necessary to have to change flights to make these dinners. Mentioning to the program that you are unable to attend do to traveling schedule is understandable.

## Mairin Jerome, PM & R

I did not drink at any pre- or post-interview dinners. I only went to one event that was focused more on drinking than food. The residents were getting pretty hammered. This turned me off from the program, mainly because it's not my scene, but I'm sure it appealed to others. I heard some stories from other applicants about getting drunk the night before an interview and being hung over on the interview day. I don't know why anyone would do this, unless you weren't interested in the program at all and just wanted to waste your time and money travelling (but getting some free drinks).

If you can, go to the interview socials. It helps give you a sense of the culture of the program. I was always impressed with programs that chose places with super delicious food. If you rsvp but can't make it for some reason, contact the residents to let them know. I waited an hour to order dinner at one event because we were waiting on one person who never showed. Most of the time, there are so many people that this isn't a big deal, but occasionally the groups will be small so just consider this and be respectful.

## Tyler van Backer, General Surgery

I never ran into the residents tossing them back quickly or wanting to go out after the social. They all understood that we had an early day the next day. At the social, I did have a couple of drinks, not more than two, though. Usually, I was barely able to finish them, though, because I was talking so much. Same thing for eating! Overall, my thoughts are that it's completely appropriate to have a beer or glass of wine. Ripping shots probably isn't appropriate, but common sense definitely applies. I waited until a resident or attending had a drink before I would order one, too.

I got asked numerous times by attendings if I had gone, if they weren't there. Others would reference our conversations from the evening before. I think it's important to go if you can for most programs. Some programs will say it "optional", but, really, it's a good time to get to know your (possibly) future co-residents. However, I did get the feeling that when people had excuses, the coordinators and residents understood and didn't hear anything negative about the applicant (not that I probably would've). If you can't make it, it's not worth canceling the interview, but definitely put in an effort to make it.

# What Do You Talk About At Socials And How Do You Really Gauge Resident Happiness?

## Samuel Austin, Anesthesia

Many people had similar questions at the pre-interview dinner. They often were related to the call schedule, the anesthesiologist-surgeon interaction, and things to do outside work. I found one of the most useful questions to ask was: "if you had the choice, would you want to match here again?" Most residents' responses were an uncanny arrangement of "yes, but there are some drawbacks". Or, "yes, and this is my favorite part about the program". I think it's a question that can alert you to a serious red-flag if the resident answers with a no (… which happened). At the same time, it is a way to indirectly frame an inquiry of what the resident came to like and dislike about the program since being in your figurative seat. Most of the responses to the straight-forward "what's your favorite aspect of the program" or "what do you like and dislike about the program" were at least semi-scripted and often wholly devoid of any real information; whereas, this question would sometimes reveal more honest sentiments. It also allowed comparison between the program you're currently at and other programs you might have already seen, as the residents often offer programs they also liked as a response to this question.

*"Have you ever seen James Bond get wasted? No? Then you probably shouldn't get hammered."*

*– Samuel Austin (on drinking at socials)*

The residents are sworn to have zero say in the way the institution ranks you (unless you're really weird one resident told us – Now that I think of it, I never heard back from that program…); however, anecdotally, I can think of an example, egregious as it may be, that (thankfully!) made its way to the program director and chair and negatively influenced this candidate's position. At this dinner, the attendees were enjoying themselves and telling jokes. Hoping to steal the spotlight, one of the candidates made a very racist joke. Even while scribing this story it makes me cringe to imagine the scene at the dinner table. Several of the residents reported the incident to the program director and you can only imagine what happened to this candidate's chances of matching to the program.

# Best / Memorable Experience

## Tyler van Backer, General Surgery

For a couple interviews, the programs went all-out and it was awesome. We had custom printed menus with gold plated lettering for one, dined at a beautiful castle-like hotel for another... For the most, part, though, they were fairly normal restaurants and a couple bars. Luckily, my embarrassing moments were mostly introducing myself twice to the same applicant or my usual level of embarrassment and nothing too extreme.

## Mairin Jerome, PM & R

I had delicious grilled octopus with grapefruit and cilantro. For a whole week of interviews right after a break-up of a 2.5-year relationship, the stress manifested as an apthous ulcer inside my upper lip that was 1cm in diameter. It was unbelievably painful and right side of my lip was really swollen. I looked like I had a botched collagen injection, and it was painful to both speak and eat, which made getting through the interview day with a big smile super tough. It took 2 weeks to go away.

## Alyssa Mendelson, General Surgery

There was some sort of lobster stew in Cleveland that I will remember for the rest of my life. Some places actually feed you, and some have like miniature appetizers that I could eat 12 of and still be starving.

I have dietary restrictions (gluten free) and definitely emailed the coordinators in advance to let them know. They always found gluten free food for me. In Chicago, we went to a pizza place and they got me my own personal gluten free pizza!

## Harold Callahan, Dermatology

I had a 4-star lunch when visiting Cleveland clinic. I had a cheese cake that moved their program up significantly in my ranking. Piece of advice: do not make fun of a city in the same state you are interviewing in. Someone in the group will have a loyalty to that place.

## Tyler van Backer, General Surgery

Early on in the interview season, applicants weren't as friendly and open with each other compared to later in the season. No one flat-out mislead me (that I know of), but later in the year, I got more honest answers about people's home programs and places where they had rotated. Even in the beginning, though, people were pretty good about discretely talking about other programs to each other. There's a sense of bonding that comes from all being in the same boat, especially towards the end when you're all tired of interviewing. It's hard to get a good representation of the program the evening before at some programs because they're designed differently (some don't allow attendings, some only let them be there for part of the evening, etc.), but talking with the residents was always really helpful. There were a few programs where the Program Director and administrators pushed their program heavily, but for the most part, it was them answering questions that we had about the program and learning about us as people (and vice-versa).

You will inevitably see someone or a couple people at multiple interviews. Your "interview buddy" can be a good resource for upcoming interviews and scouting out other places, discretely, of course. There were a couple of people who I met who realized they were heading to the same interview and ended up driving together, too.

## Alyssa Mendelson, General Surgery

If there were students who either went to the medical school at the program or who rotated there, I definitely asked them what they thought of the place. I never had anyone try to mislead me. People were honest in saying "yes, I love this place, I'm trying to stay here", or "meh, it depends on what you're looking for in a program." They also had insight as to how residents interacted with students – this was important to me because I'm interested in education!

## Samuel Austin, Anesthesia

Most people who spent a month at the program were happy to give their advice, often unsolicited. Use your best judgment with these people. Gunners get interviews, too. So it's true that the person spewing advice may be misleading you; however, nearly everyone I met seemed kind, honest, and cool. It was actually really cool to meet and get to know the other applicants. I still talk to some of the people I met on interviews.

# 11

## INTERVIEW DAY

*The Ultimate Purpose, Asking Questions, Being Caught Off Guard, Post-Interview Communication*

# The Ultimate Purpose of Interviews

### Whitney Alduron, Anesthesia

I'm not sure what the purpose of interviews is, but in my mind I tell myself that it is to decide whether they want to work with me for the next 3 to 4 years, and if they think I'm a (relatively) normal person. It is definitely very challenging to decide whether you want to spend your residency at a program after only a few hours at the hospital and meeting a select few faculty or residents.

Overall it comes down to the feeling that you get from the location and the people that you interact with. It's difficult to describe in words, but you just know whether this is a place you want to be or not.

## Tyler van Backer, General Surgery

From the program's standpoint, I honestly think that it was for programs to see if they could work with me for 5-7 years or if I would be a completely awful investment of time. For me, I really used it to see if I could stand to be there for 5-7 years of my life and if I could see myself being happy there.

> *"One thing I noticed that I needed to watch out for was that I began basing the program off of the other applicants. I started thinking "will these people be friends of mine?""*
>
> *-Whitney Alduron*

For the most part, I felt like I had a mediocre amount of information compared to where I did rotations and my home institution. Unfortunately, that's the way it goes, though because you can't rotate at all the hospitals. Don't get me wrong, you'll get more Power-Points on case logs and "why our program is unique" than you can stay awake for, but I really wanted to know if the program was good, if it could get me to where I want to go, and if I would 'enjoy' myself there. Those things don't really come across well in PowerPoint, but I was able to talk with more residents and go with some gut feelings about programs to formulate my rank list. I would also suggest second look days if you can't decide or want more information.

## Cameron Smith, Internal Medicine

For internal medicine, I think the interviews are designed to see if the interviewee will fit in with the cohort of residents and attendings. They want to make sure they are selecting people that are able to communicate well with other physicians and with their patients.

## Alyssa Mendelson, General Surgery

To make sure you're not an asshole.

## Samuel Austin, Anesthesia

The ultimate purpose of the interview is to get an idea of your understanding of the specialty and your interpersonal skills. The last thing a program wants is someone who leaves partway through. Well, second to last, maybe. First, they don't want a diddler or a serial killer. That's bad publicity.

## Mairin Jerome, PM & R

The majority of programs cared about who I am as a person. They appeared interested in my travels, volunteer experiences, and my work with underserved populations. Interviewers asked frequently about my interests outside of medicine. Their overall goal is to make sure they match people who fit in well, work hard, and are easy to work with.

## Cameron Smith, Internal Medicine

Expect any and all questions on your interview day. Some of the more common questions that I got were:

1. Tell us about a challenging experience and how you reacted
2. What is one of your strengths/weaknesses
3. Who is one of your role models or who is your hero
4. Why do you want to enter the field you are applying for
5. Some open ended questions (tell me about yourself...)

# All About Interview Day

## Calvin Barber, Anesthesia

I think I got a fair representation of programs, but you know they're on their best behavior. They're all trying to sell - everyone gives you a folder with handouts, gifts, a lot of places give you flash drives with their logo, some places gave me mugs and leather bound notebooks with the school monogram on the book. I mean all the programs give the same presentation; they will all do the same as you are doing in your personal statement. They will try to answer the things they know are going to be asked. If they're weak in a particular area, they will address that in their presentation. They will all tell you that you're a great candidate, and they're a great program, and you should make beautiful medicine together.

Nearly everywhere asked the behavioral questions like, "when you witnessed a medical error…" all that kind of stuff. What is your greatest weakness? Those kinds of things were very common - I think they are ridiculous questions. Everyone knows they are coming, everyone's prepared an answer. What will that tell you? Even worse than that, I think maybe twice in all my interviews I was asked academic questions. What is the point of that? You have so much data on what I know factually, scores, everything from my school from the pre-clinical coursework to every rotation, you should know academically where I stand. What does it tell you if I get that question wrong? Right, nothing at all. I don't know why anyone would choose to ask those questions.

Speaking briefly about interviews, my attitude toward interviews was very much like doing a chat show. I came in with a couple of questions I expected that they were going to ask me and I had answers prepared for those fairly straightforward ones. I also came in with a willingness to talk about anything at all, to really try to engage the person interviewing me in a conversation, and not worry about where those conversations went. I was willing to talk about everything from end-of-life decision-making to whether I personally consider Halle Berry to be sexy, as opposed to beautiful. I did talk about both of those things at different interviews.

Your goal in an interview is to seem like someone who would be cool to be around 3 o'clock in the morning when you've just been called in, the crisis is about to happen. You want to be someone who's going to be fun to hang out with. I think that makes you a very appealing candidate.

## Alyssa Mendelson, General Surgery

My first few interviews I was super nervous, and I definitely tried to answer questions based on what I thought the interviewer wanted to hear. This was stupid. It made me overanalyze everything and panic. When it comes down to it, answering questions honestly and communicating in your own way is important. If a program doesn't like you for you, you're going to have some real problems later down the line.

A program could have a ton of great departments, research experiences etc., but if you get a weird vibe, listen to it. You can really get a good feel for the attendings and what the program values based off of the interviews. If they want to drill you in front of other students on a panel interview, to me that says "we're a really competitive, cut-throat program. The person sitting next to you is a colleague, not a friend." That was not the type of program I was looking for. Others were really pleasant conversations about whatever topics came up.

I personally was looking for an academic program with a variety of opportunities for research, a work-life balance, and a supportive group of attendings. Little details like the electronic medical record (EMR) or number of ICU months during PGY-2 year were important, but not "big-picture" enough for me to gauge whether I would really be happy there.

I felt like the research experiences were easy to gauge. You can usually find these on the website, or just ask the research residents at the pre-interview reception or during the interview day.

Resident happiness was tough to gauge. At a couple interviews, I only met close to four residents when some of these programs had 10+ residents per year. Where were the rest of them? All working? Didn't want to show up?

At other interviews, I met a lot of residents, and I could gauge how well they got along by the interactions/conversations they had with each other when they thought no one was watching. They would hug, laugh, joke, etc. Also, they would be really honest about the strengths and weaknesses of the program, and had all sorts of concrete examples of activities they would do with one another outside the hospital. The pre-interview reception is definitely the best time to gauge these things. And again, a lot of this is just gut feeling!

> *"Every program will tell you that you're a great candidate, and they're a great program, and you should make beautiful medicine together."*
>
> *-Calvin Barber*

## Burt Johnson, Urology

Interview day is pretty basic. Be professional but be relaxed. In my mind the actual interview day was less about quizzing you and more about getting to know you as a person. Again it comes back to trying to put yourself in the position of the interviewers and the program, really considering what their motivations are. I think they just wanted figure out who you are; can they spend time with you for five years? Are you a weirdo?

I'm not sure that there is much more that you can glean from 15 to 20 minute interactions with someone other than their personality, their attitude, and their interest. The baseline assumption is that if you already have been invited to interview, you are academically qualified and interesting enough.

For example, in urology, most programs interviewed about 40 applicants out of a pool of anywhere between 250 and 350 applications they received. If you've been invited to interview, this should put you in the mindset that both parties are interviewing each other rather than you are being interviewed by them. In my experience, it was a very friendly more conversational atmosphere where people were just trying to get to know each other.

You need to know your resume back and front. You need to be able to talk about anything you put on the resume. This goes back to my comments in the ERAS application section where I personally decided to be a little bit more conservative about what I put on my CV. I wanted to be very comfortable talking about anything on my resume, and the interviewers wouldn't lead me on tangential conversations.

Be prepared for two of the fundamental interview questions.

Why do you want to do urology?

Why do you want to come to our program?

You need to have solid, confident, and logical answers to these. It doesn't need to be something crazy and elaborate, but it can be a something as simple as,

'I think is a top-notch program with great research that I'd love to be a part of. You train great surgeons, my significant other has family here, and we'd really be happy in this city.'

Simple answers for programs you are actually interested in, you'll have to be more creative for programs that you're not so high on. No one's looking for anything fancy, just looking for honesty and directness.

Save all your nitty-gritty logistical and detailed questions for the residents because you don't want to waste a question like that during limited time with an attending. Residents are less judgmental, and they know what students and applicants really care about. It wasn't so long ago when they were on the interview trail themselves.

Other questions:

Tell me about yourself!

What are your strengths and weaknesses?

What are your goals?

Where do you see yourself in five years? 10 years?

Make a list of top 10 questions and just prepare answers for them. You've memorized more during 4 years of school. The reality is that most applicants will have prepared answers for that, and if you're not ready to answer with tact and brevity than you may hurt yourself. Be polished.

What I did was simply to identify 5 to 10 common questions I thought would be asked prior to interviews, and I just typed up a strategy of talking points and the message that I wanted to get across about myself and work that into the answers. I didn't memorize things verbatim, but I just knew going in what my ideas were and where I wanted to lead the conversation. 'Tell me about yourself' is a classic opener and you should view it as a gift to be asked this question. It is a quick way to tell your story and allows you to direct the conversation on your terms. A strong answer to this question allows you to take control of the interview, and that's what you really want.

Assessing resident happiness and quality of life is difficult, but hopefully from interacting with the residents you can gather information. Programs that have a priority on residency training and education often display this by shutting down their clinics and operating rooms for the entire interview day. This represents a significant financial investment. However, while this does denote a commitment to residency training, every program that did this was very keen to mention it as well. On the flipside there were programs that only had the research residents at the interview day. This gives you an incredibly skewed view of what a residency life is like. Research residents have very cushy schedules and are typically very happy and have very few clinical duties. This unrealistically or at least subconsciously gives you the impression that their quality of life is excellent. It also shows you that they either don't think it's valuable for you to talk to the current residents or they rely on their residents so heavily that they can't take them out of work. Resident attendance at the pre or post-interview social is also a nice marker for how much energy residents have after work.

One question I felt like every applicant asked on interview trail was [to residents],

"Do you spend time together outside of the hospital?"

And during my first few interviews, I certainly asked this question because I thought it might be a view into the culture at the residency program. When I was at UConn, about halfway through the season, we were riding in one of the chief's cars, and he basically said how silly of a question that is. Basically, every resident works together for 60 to 80 hours a week and that's usually enough time to be spending with each other. After a long day in OR, spending more time with those they see every single day doesn't sound so appetizing.

## Alyssa Mendelson, General Surgery

I had a few programs ask me ethical questions – physician assisted suicide, etc. I also had a behavioral interview question, "Describe a time when you interacted with a resident or attending and you disagreed with a decision they made. What did you do?"

My advice would be to be laid back with these, they aren't supposed to make you nervous, they are supposed to make you think. I honestly think half the time they don't care what your answer is – they are judging you off your ability to stay calm and think through an uncomfortable situation. Don't just make up an answer, take a few seconds or a minute and really think of an example from your clinical years. Alternatively, do some thinking before you go on interviews so you have a couple of these scenarios in your back pocket. The interviewers are smart, and they can tell when you fabricating a story to tell them what they want to hear.

Also, smile a lot. Psychologically it makes you and the interviewer feel more at ease.

Also, if you are from a state where there are interesting things going on in the news – i.e. healthcare reform, weird politics, etc. - try to stay updated on the topic. I'm from Vermont and at the time the state was trying to implement universal health care. This came up multiple times at interviews, both as interview questions and as small talk. Be sure to tread carefully on topics in terms or sharing your opinions, you never know what side of the fence your interviewer is on.

## G. Michael Krauthamer, Emergency Medicine

So let's say you've secured a few interviews. Rule number one is fairly obvious, don't be late! (it goes without saying that no-showing is really poor form). Walking in late is embarrassing, and you may be asked during an interview why you were late which puts you in the awkward position of having to explain your apparent lack of professionalism (I speak from personal experience). If you are going to be late because you got lost or your flight is delayed, call the program administrator early in the morning before the interview day starts.

Prior to interviews, anticipate possible questions and contemplate your responses. Initially I did not do this, and some questions really caught me off guard the first time around, causing me to stumble for answers and generally appear awkward. After a couple of these experiences, I talked to a friend of mine who works as a recruiter for a large law firm in Manhattan. She was dumbfounded to learn that I hadn't actually rehearsed answers to common interview questions such as, "why do you want to come to this program," and "what do you think will be the hardest thing for you during residency," and "Describe a situation where you've had to act as a leader, deal with conflict, faced adversity etc…"

Your answers should be specific without raising red flags (another lesson learned the hard way—I think my unpracticed answer to the "facing adversity" question was something embarrassingly adolescent, like I didn't get along with my mom as a kid, or something equally inane. On the other hand my practiced answer was that as an African-American man, I had of course contended, at different times, with the adversity that attends racism, and that these experiences ultimately served to codify my commitment to providing the highest quality care to all patients while making me particularly sensitive to the needs of historically underserved individuals.)

There will be some of you (myself included) that have a change of heart and specialty late in the process. Figure out a salient explanation for your last minute change and be prepared to articulate this to interviewers. I tended to be frank with my interviewers about my interests in psychiatry but emphasized that what I like most about psychiatry was the "emergent" situations; that this was the realization which led me to initially consider emergency medicine, and that since completing my sub-internships in Emergency Medicine, I could confidently say that I had made the right choice.

Similarly, although I had substantial research background, most of it was in psychiatry research. Occasionally interviewers would ask, "Won't it be hard for you to give up your research," to which I responded, "My past experience has provided me with excellent experience in devising interesting and clinically relevant research questions, and I am excited to bring these skills to bear as an Emergency Medicine doctor." The point is, know that you will be challenged on your choice of specialty; more so if it is obvious from your application that you made the decision late in your medical school career, so you should be prepared to defend your choices.

The fact remains that you will have bad interviews and good interviews, and you will get better with practice; While I foolishly did not prepare for the predictable interview questions, I did specifically scheduled a few early interviews at programs that I was less interested in, in order to get practice with the interview process before interviewing at programs I really hoped to rank highly.

## Dena Darby, Family Medicine

There are some interview days that won't go well. Right off the bat, you may feel that you don't fit in or one of their representatives may leave a poor impression. I never left an interview day early, but I did leave at least one knowing that I wouldn't even rank that program. While I do think it is good etiquette to cancel an interview day at a program you have no interest in, I would advise against leaving the day early which can come off as rude and insulting. Word gets around. On the other hand, take the moments of discomfort with a grain of salt – there are misunderstandings and one person does not represent the whole institution.

## Mairin Jerome, PM & R

I liked asking interviewers how they ended up in PM & R. Most seemed excited to talk about it. In terms of specific questions about programs, I liked asking about the diversity within patient populations and demographics.

I particularly wanted to find out about procedure volume. There was a big distinction between programs in this program. All PM & R programs can say they have 200+ EMGs, because that is an ACGME requirement, but all other procedures will be logged as well. Senior residents at some programs could give me specific numbers (i.e. "I have done 150+ axial spine procedures myself' or "I am a PGY2 and over the last 6 months I have probably done 30 joint injections." I found that at some programs, if I asked a program director about specific numbers of procedures, I got a non-specific answer.

## Tyler van Backer, General Surgery

Tell me about yourself was the most common question I got. I loved this question because it was always first, and it completely puts you in the driver's seat for where you want to take the interview. I quickly went over where I grew up, very very briefly why surgery/medicine, which highlighted some achievements, and then extracurriculars in college that steered me toward surgery. Briefly, I included a few activities in medical school (intra and extramural- remember, it's important to show you're more than just a student and unless they're blinded, they have your CV). Other good questions I was asked were more silly, like 'what's your theme song'.

Strategically, I knew that I wanted to throw in a couple "easy" interviews in the beginning. At a certain point, it's beyond your control, but if possible try to have a couple under your belt before you go into what you think are your top choices. I learned a great amount about my application and how to interview (even having done mock interviews with my home institution) in the first couple interviews. There are also only so many questions that usually get answered, so having a well-oiled, yet not obviously rehearsed, answer is a good thing to have for your favorite programs.

> *"The last thing a program wants is someone who leaves partway through. Well, second to last, maybe. First, they don't want a diddler or a serial killer. That's bad publicity."*
>
> *-Samuel Austin*

For programs, it was a must that the residents get along. Surgery (and most residencies, from what I gather) are long hours and hard enough, so you really need to like the people you'll be seeing every day. Same goes for attending surgeons. If programs had high turnover, I would cautiously ask the residents what were the circumstances. I'm somewhat interested in cardiac surgery, so an ability to be exposed to that field was also up on my list. I tried to make sure that the programs that I interviewed at were placing people into fellowships that I was considering. I also made sure that they had residents graduating into practice too proving technical competency after a standard residency. Another consideration was the boards passing rate (ABS has the five year rates for all the programs on their website). Talking to residents and looking through program websites got me most of the information, and then I asked program directors or attendings for the rest during the interview or evening prior. Oddly enough, I also placed a certain amount of importance on what electronic medical record (EMR) the hospital used. Paper charts with Soarian? No, thanks. EPIC was music to my ears. It seems kind of shallow and unimportant, but as a resident we'll be spending more hours than I care to count on the computer and entering orders/writing notes/rounding. The better the EMR, the more efficient I can be.

I took notes during the presentations, occasionally, of things that I liked or didn't like. I also tried to write down what we talked about during an interview immediately afterwards so I could use that information for a thank you note. I used my gut for the three tiers of programs on my list (would love to go to any, would be happy at these, and would rather match than not match, but not my favorites) and then my notes to move programs around within each category.

## Dena Darby, Family Medicine

### "Made in Japan"

You will make some mistakes – you will say awkward things, make ill-received jokes. Don't let these ruin your day. Move on and present your best self. I was in a program director's office, where he had many pieces of Japanese memorabilia on the walls – photos, awards, etc. I shared with him that I was "Made in Japan" – in fact, that is where my parents lived when I was conceived. This is how my interview began. After that, it actually went pretty well.

# Do You Have Any Questions???

At every interview, you will be afforded the opportunity to ask any question you wish. At a certain point, every interviewee has inevitably run out of questions to ask. These are there suggestions and stories…

## Whitney Alduron, Anesthesia

One of my favorite questions I liked asking was "what is your favorite aspect of the program?" I think a lot of students ask the negative "what would you change about the program?" (or some iteration of that), but I think by putting a positive spin on your questions makes it well-received. Obviously different programs have different interview styles. Some ask a lot of behavioral questions such as "Tell me about a situation where you were made to feel inadequate, how did you deal with it" or "Tell me about a time you were put into a leadership position, how did you handle that?" Others ask arbitrary and, in my mind, stupid questions such as "What is your spirit animal?" "What is your favorite color?"

One of the most memorable interviews outright stated,

"We are not going to ask you any questions because we have already read your application and decided you would be a great fit here, and so this is your time to ask us questions to find out if this is the right program for you."

That was probably the most challenging interview day because to have five back-to-back 20 minute interviews that you need to fill with questions becomes tedious.

## Alyssa Mendelson, General Surgery

This is seriously the worst part about interviews. You will get all of your questions answered in the first hour, and then everyone for the rest of the day would ask you if you had any more questions. Don't scream "NO I DON'T, STOP ASKING ME THAT," like you want to. I typically would start asking people what their favorite part of the program was (cheesy) but then occasionally they would say something that could prompt another question. "My favorite part of the program is our interactions with residents. We really feel like a community here." "Oh? What types of social gatherings do faculty and residents have outside the hospital…" etc. etc.

Also, if I couldn't come up with a question I said "The residents and faculty here have been so great! Everyone has been very honest and helpful in answering all of my questions. One question I did have that got answered already was blah, blah, blah, which was really impressive to me." This gives your interviewer something to talk about (or not, if they don't have anything additional to add) without you actually having to come up with a new question. Then, you don't sound like an idiot who knows nothing about the program or doesn't care about the program.

## Burt Johnson, Urology

A challenging part of interviews is the dreaded time when the interviewer asks you, "do you have any questions?" Some interviewers will give you five minutes at the end, some will be one minute at the end, and some interviews will consist only of your questions. Having 3, 4, 5 questions to ask in your back pocket is just as important as having answers to the 5 most common questions.

Prior to medical school, I had interviewed for other jobs so I had a little interview practice and had received some advice before. One of the best tips I got was at my first real job interview. I had never interviewed before and was a total rookie. At the end of the interview, the interviewer said to me that I'm not getting the job, but here are some things you can work on for interviewing. The one item that stuck with me was 'you need to ask the interviewer about their life and their experiences.' This serves two purposes:

1) You learn about the interviewer, their personality, priorities

2) People love talking about themselves. What they remember after the interview is their overall feeling of how it went and subconsciously when people talk

about themselves, they have a positive feeling about the experience. Use that to your advantage.

One question that I always had at the ready was "tell me about how you got to this position and what brought you specifically to this program?" I felt like this was a good example of an open ended question that would let the interviewer talk. From there I would just pick out some things they mentioned and ask more about it. I was less interested in asking logistical questions about the program and what they thought the strengths were because realistically those were all going to be canned answers and wouldn't give me much information in any way.

There were a couple occasions where I asked my two or three open-ended questions and the interviewer answered them curtly. I had no more questions and I simply said, 'I think I have a pretty good idea of the program and talked a lot to the residents and have no other specific questions for you.'

## Samuel Austin, Anesthesia

My first interview got awkward when I ran out of questions. I started asking the faculty member about his schedule, to which I received one word responses that left me scrambling to find another question about his schedule to ask. I wish there were a recording of these tortuous two minutes because it was probably a hilarious scene. Learn from my mistake and come ready.

Ask what you want to know. I got good responses from "what about this program makes you most proud?" and "if you had unlimited resources and people to help, what's something you might change about the program?" When in a pinch, ask about the interviewer's story as to how he or she got to the place you're interviewing, or how they chose the specialty, etc…

## G. Michael Krauthamer, Emergency Medicine

Sometimes you will get asked ridiculous and seemingly irrelevant questions ("what musical artist would you listen to before and after a shift;" "Who's on first?"). These appear to be intended to show how laid back your interviewer is, but will actually just feel awkward and contrived. Just do your best to laugh these off and roll with these types of questions.

Ultimately, try to direct the conversation towards topics about which you are passionate, and ideally, interview toward highlighting your strengths. Try your best to convey your passion for medicine and your chosen specialty. It sounds cliché to say this but mostly, try to be yourself; the interview provides the opportunity for programs to get to know you in the flesh. Many directors said, "If you are here, you've already passed our test, and we want you, so the interview day is for you to decide if you want to be here." While this may be an exaggeration, the point is well taken—if programs are not genuinely interested in you, they won't invite you for an interview thus in a sense, once you've been invited to an interview, the spot is yours to choose (or lose).

## Dena Darby, Family Medicine

**It is ALL part of the interview**

At one interview day in the Northeast, the applicants waited in the break room with two residents between interviews. It was presented as a time to ask questions and hear the resident perspective – a valuable opportunity. We grabbed some coffee and water and sat around the table. There were about five applicants, and the residents introduced themselves and said, "Don't worry, this isn't part of the interview, just a chance to chat." We all smiled at each other. A short silence followed, then one of the residents turned to the first applicant and asked, "So what do you think some of your strengths are, and what would you bring to our program?" He looked surprised, the same way that I felt. I was glad that I sat about four people down. The poor guy stumbled through an answer, clearly caught off-guard. Down the line of applicants, we had slightly better answers prepared due to having a few extra minutes. This example just reminded me that it is all part of the interview – from the first email to the coordinator to your follow-up thank you notes. They are paying attention to what you're wearing, how you communicate, how you use the downtime. Don't let this make you nervous; you should still be yourself and try to relax, but just remember that it is all part of it.

## Mairin Jerome, PM & R

1. What type of support it there for research?

2. How much hands-on exposure is there? How much autonomy do residents have?

3. It is okay to not ask any more questions. I would just say, all of the questions I had so far had been answered.

## Tyler van Backer, General Surgery

Always have questions. Always. There's no excuse for not having a question because you can re-ask questions to get different people's opinions. Sometimes I prefaced questions with 'I like to ask this of everyone to get different viewpoints on…' When I was stuck, I went with 'how will the program look different in 5-7 years when I'm a chief resident?' or 'what qualities do you look for in a resident that I haven't satisfactorily demonstrated?' Both are rather direct questions, but show that you really have a vested interest in vetting the program and are taking it seriously. When my interviewer was just me asking questions, I would ask about how proficient they felt the residents were technically, with patient care, or what they liked about living in the area.

## Cameron Smith, Internal Medicine

I tried to ask questions that were specific to the program. I would listen attentively during the presentations given by residents or the program director, and come up with questions that show that I was interested in specific aspects of the program. Of course, I did have some go-to questions that I would ask of most programs, which were the following:

1. What is the biggest weakness of your program?
2. Is there a mentoring program at this institution?
3. Is there a sense of resident autonomy at this program?
4. What is the EMR that is used here?
5. What specific research opportunities are there available to residents?
6. What is the structure of the clinic?

I would advise to schedule the first 1-2 interviews at programs where you are least interested in. That way, you do not feel as much pressure to do well, and can get a hang of the structure of interviews and the types of questions that are asked of you.

It's difficult to figure out the entirety of a residency program from a half-day interview. I recommend talking to the residents as much as possible, and maybe even getting a few email addresses and staying in touch with them throughout the interview process to ask any questions that may come up at a later time.

The most important thing you get out of an interview is the feel for the program. You want to experience the vibe at that particular place, and get an idea of the culture. Ask yourself if you would be able to spend long hours with these types of people, and in that specific environment.

Don't get distracted by the bells and whistles regarding research and curriculum, your priority should be to assess the program's fit for your personality. I personally was looking for a place that offered ample research opportunities, freedom for residents to make clinical decisions, and a place that offered a varying degree of pathology. At the same time, I wanted to make sure I would end up at a place where residents were happy and enjoyed what they do. It was pretty evident to me which programs the residents enjoyed, based on how passionately they spoke about it during the interview day.

# Caught Off Guard

## Dena Darby, Family Medicine

### Different kinds of interviews and being ready for all of them

There are different tones of interview and different interviewers out there – most of my interviews were "what are you interested in?" and "what do you do for fun?", but there was the occasional, more challenging "tell me about a difficult situation that you encountered with a colleague and how you handled it". Particularly in Family Medicine, the conversations were mostly about why we both love Family Medicine (I did not find that discussion to be straining). The rapid-fire "tell me about a difficult situation" and "what are your weaknesses" caught me off guard. Even at the same institution, there is huge variability within the interviewers. You can let them set the tone of the interview, and never be afraid to ask your interviewer an open-ended question if you need a break from talking.

## Alyssa Mendelson, General Surgery

Some people are rude - program directors, faculty, residents. Just expect early on that it's going to happen. Be patient and don't be rude back.

I definitely was more at ease during my later interviews. I did not schedule any of my favorite programs first for that reason. I knew I would want to get my feet wet with a couple and get a feel for the process. I'm really glad I did that.

That being said, I was SUPER TIRED for my last three. My motivation was low, I was exhausted from traveling, I was exhausted from answering the same questions over and over again, and I was exhausted of asking the same questions over and again. Keep that in mind. The number one program on my rank list was in my last three interviews…

## Burt Johnson, Urology

I'm not sure that anything in specific caught me off guard while I was interviewing, but I will say that as an interviewee you should expect to be tested a little bit.

> *"Best question I was asked: if there were literally no need for medicine anymore – everyone is completely healthy – what would you do? I told them I'd love to play music for a living. It was a toss-up between rock star and rally car racer, but let's be honest: rockers get all the chicks."*
>
> *-Samuel Austin*

I ran into one situation where interviewers tried to get under my skin a little. The interviews were 15 to 20 minute 1-on-1 interviews with one to three interviewers. The interviewers asked me why I wanted to go to their program and after I told them, they said "no you really want to go to program x." I just tried to keep my cool and be calm - simply just reiterate why I thought their program was excellent. They repeatedly tried to hammer their previous point. This was a rare example of intentionally or unintentionally getting under your skin to test you and see if you can handle pressure situations.

I can partly understand this, but in my mind it is a foolish tactic from an interviewer/program standpoint. You may find out applicants that are weak under pressure and may crumble, and that's great. However, the people that thrive or withstand the onslaught will have a negative experience. Applicants worth their salt know that they have leverage in this experience, and it really is a bilateral interview. So if as the interviewer you try and test them with irritating questions, the interviewees will recognize that the priorities of the program and applicant are not aligned.

One experience I will share is about having a chip on your shoulder. I personally didn't go to medical school at a big-name program. I went to a smaller New England medical school and status-wise was not on the same level as the powerhouse schools in the country. What I didn't realize until one of interviewers flat out told me was to never be defensive about going to a smaller school and being interviewed alongside folks from big-name institutions. To him, it's more of an accomplishment to go to a small school with limited resources and accomplish more than to go to the big name and not get as much done. In talking with this one interviewer at Cornell, unexpectedly, I sort of turned a chip on my shoulder into a strength that I could advertise in future interviews. So if you're in a similar position don't immediately assume that programs think less of you. They are interested in what you've done and what you will do. After all, they invited you for an interview.

## Whitney Alduron, Anesthesia

I think one of the best questions I was asked that completely caught me off guard and I did not have an answer for was "so what do we need to do to get you to come here?" I have been so conditioned to ask that question myself that I did not have an answer when it was flipped on me and I have to admit laughing and saying "I don't know" was probably not the best.

Sometimes I took notes during the PowerPoint presentations, but more to keep me awake then to provide any sort of information. Looking back, if they did not give me a USB with the PowerPoint, I would've forgotten the key information if I had not written it down.

I don't think I was asked any illegal questions, the only question that was perhaps borderline was "Is your boyfriend planning to move here with you?"

## Tyler van Backer, General Surgery

A couple questions caught me off-guard, despite having prepared (I thought) for them. I was asked why I only passed an away rotation, which I managed to pull out some answer about it being my first rotation as a fourth year and I was transitioning between being an interpreter to a manager (somehow remembered those stages of learning from somewhere!) Quick recovery. Another that caught me off guard was to name three people I would like to meet/have over for dinner and one person to kill (without any moral/ethical/legal implications) and why.

I too had the 'what's your spirit animal' question. Nothing made me laugh out loud because it was inherently funny, but I started smirking at the repetitiveness of questions by the end of interview season.

Going to be late? It's all about communication. Flight gets delayed? Stuck in on the interstate because they shut down the highway? Just call the program administrator and let him or her know. Obviously, it looks bad if you waltz in late to the interview (especially if you were there the night before…), but it's just about being respectful of their time/energy- just communicate what's going on.

## Mairin Jerome, PM & R

This is pretty embarrassing, but I will share so others don't make this same ridiculous mistake. I went into interview season with the attitude of using the interviews to see whether or not I liked the program and if I would want to go there. So, at one prestigious institution, a chief resident interviewing me asked me point blank why I wanted to go to that program and why I wanted to live in that city. Oddly, this took me off guard because I was thinking, "well, I don't even know yet if I for sure want to come here or if I want to live in this city." Even if this is really what you think, have an answer ready as though this is your first choice. I totally botched this even though there were a million reasons why I thought this was a great program and why I liked the city. Again, it was one of my first interviews and I was nervous.

## Cameron Smith, Internal Medicine

The question that caught me most off guard was to describe one confrontation I had with someone in my life and how I dealt with it. I tend to be a non-confrontational person to begin with, so it took me about 20-30 seconds to really think of something.

# Questions You Wished You'd Asked ...

## Alyssa Mendelson, General Surgery

This would have been awkward to ask, but I found out one of the programs I interviewed at got a citation for "Fear of intimidation" by residents and students. #scary

## Tyler van Backer, General Surgery

If I had to do it again, I would have tailored my questions more towards each program and then had a set of questions that I also made sure to ask to each program. My notes are sometimes comparing apples to oranges, which is frustrating when it comes to deciding the difference between number 3 and 4 or 8 and 9 on the rank list.

# Post-Interview Communication

## Alyssa Mendelson, General Surgery

I started off hand-writing a thank you note to every person who interviewed me. This was anywhere from 3-7 thank you notes per program. I would try to get them out in a week. As I progressed through the interview process, I would only write 1-2 to people I really connected with. If I connected with no one, I would just send one to the program director. For two programs that I didn't like much at all, I didn't write any. Do your best to write some thank you notes.

I've heard hand-written is better than email. My thank you cards were blank ivory and simple. None of the fru-fru squirrels holding an acorn with "thank you" written in a bubble above their heads.

My template was:

*"Dear Dr. Important Surgeon,*

*I wanted to thank you for the invitation to interview at the University of Surgery. Your program is truly exceptional in the realms of academic excellence, resident education and quality patient care.*

*Personally, I appreciated "insert personal conversation piece here".*

*The University of Surgery will certainly be among my top choices (first choice, etc.) It would be an absolute honor to work with your faculty and house staff as I embark on my surgical training. Thank you again for the opportunity to share my experience and interest, and I hope to speak with you again in the near future.*

*Best,*

*Alyssa Mendelson"*

Most of my programs said they would not be sending out letters after interviews as they "respect the Match process." However, I have received at least one personalized letter encouraging me to please please please strongly consider their program. The letter was so sweet, and so detailed about every interaction anyone had with me on my interview day that I have a hard time believing they are bullshitting me. That being said, I honestly don't know what role these letters play.

## G. Michael Krauthamer, Emergency Medicine

The jury is split on sending thank you cards after interviews. Here is what I did: I emailed all of the places I interviewed and thanked them for inviting me. I then set up second look visits at my top three programs. Finally, after my second look visits, I sent follow-up emails to the program directors at these programs reiterating my strong interest. I tried to be concise but specific about why I was interested in a given program. In more than one case, the program director emailed me back thanking me, and more or less telling me that they would rank me highly. It seems important to emphasize that the second look visit is invaluable in this regard for demonstrating your interest in a program. I was told that programs fear ranking candidates who will not rank them, so letting a program really know your interest can only help your chances.

## Samuel Austin, Anesthesia

I wrote thank you notes to everyone with whom I interviewed. And by notes I mean emails. In those emails I thanked them for the opportunity to visit the program and commented on specific things we talked about during the interview. Many of these emails weren't responded to, but it's all good.

I was contacted by programs informing that I was "ranked to match", in their vernacular. One program called very early on which made for an awkward conversation, though their program was my favorite. I really felt like I should reciprocate by telling them they were my #1, I honestly couldn't say it at the time because I wasn't sure what other programs would feel like. I received emails at the end of the interview season from a few more programs, which went more or less like, "this is why you should come here, rank us highly." Others were more generic from chief residents asking if there were additional questions I had. At the end of the interview season I received another phone call from my #1 program. All-in-all, it's nice to get these emails and calls; however, I had a hard time actually putting much stake in them. You should rank where you want to go, not where you think will be a sure thing. Anyone can say anything and the proof is in the pudding on Match Day.

Finally, you need to be honest when replying to this sort of communication. Programs have likely been burnt by people saying they're ranking them #1 in the past, and the same is likely true of applicants. Use your words carefully and wisely – medicine is a very small world and dishonesty will be remembered. If they're not your #1, don't say that they are; that said, you also don't need to volunteer that they aren't.

I didn't have the PD of my home program call my top choice, but there were other faculty in the department familiar with that program who went to bat for me.

## Burt Johnson, Urology

I thought this might come back and burn me at some point, but I did not send thank you letters to every program I interviewed at. The first program I interviewed at was Dartmouth, and their program director explicitly said she did not want thank you letters because it's a waste of time. They don't add anything to your application. I personally did not write thank you letter to every program, but I did write thank you emails to programs that really got me excited. This may have been a mistake, but I ended up matching at great program anyway. In fact I didn't even write thank you letters or thank you emails to the program I ended up matching at. However, I did make an attempt to take a second look, and they said don't worry about it, "message heard loud and clear." I think there's a fairly reasonable chance that if you did a randomized controlled trial with thank you notes versus no contact you would find out that writing notes maybe doesn't matter as much as people think they do. However, in terms of cost/benefit, it's probably safer to write the notes.

A game goes on about telling programs where you're going to rank them. Conventionally, you tell your first choice program that you will be ranking them first. Keep in mind that if you do tell the program you better commit to that, barring any life altering problems. If you tell the program you will rank them number one, they rank you number one, and you match elsewhere, they know that you didn't rank them first. Remember that residency training is not the end of the road – you will need to find a job eventually, and in particularly small fields people talk to each other a lot, and they remember these things. Forget about getting a job at the place you misled, and potentially many others. If you're not 100% sure which is #1, don't tell them. The other item is that sometimes people suggest telling your number two and number three programs that you are going to rank them 'very highly.' I feel like these are all items that are well understood when it comes to reading between the lines as far as the program's interpretation of your communication.

I personally did not tell any program that I would rank them number one for two reasons. The first was practical: up until the last day before I had submit my rank list I was going back and forth between two programs. The second reason was that playing this game in my mind is really an attempt to circumvent the match process.

The other item to address is second looks. Every program will tell you that second looks (when you visit a program at some point after interview day to re-look at the program) are not required and that they are only for your personal education about how things operate at their residency program. This may be true, but they take it into account as another sign of your interest in their program. If you really like a program or really want to find out more about it go for a second look. It may not benefit you at all, but the odds are that it probably won't hurt you. Programs like Penn were pretty obvious that if you wanted to match there, you had to do a second look. This was the prevailing wisdom on the interview trail (at least for urology).

As for programs contacting me after the interviews, it was actually quite rare. I got an occasional friendly email, but I didn't receive any illegal offers or communication from programs. Additionally, I didn't have anyone make phone calls for me on my behalf although this is legitimate and can really be in your favor to do.

## Dena Darby, Family Medicine

I sent the golden "you are my number one" message to my top program's director. I received a nice message back, which I found encouraging, until my friend and classmate told me the story of an applicant who communicated with their number one and was misled. This applicant told their number one program about their intentions to rank them first, and actually received a response saying the program would rank this applicant number one as well. When Match Day arrived, the applicant DID NOT match at that program. Since he ranked them number one, the only explanation is that the program did not rank him number one in return as they stated. Granted this story is third-hand, but this is not the only story of this kind that I have heard. What keeps us from lying to programs? Hopefully, an intrinsic moral compass, but you could also argue for maintaining your reputation. What keeps programs from lying to us? Possibly the same moral compass, or simply reputation maintenance. You may receive encouraging emails from programs that seem almost probing as they let you know how interested they are in having you work with them. Be honest in your communication, be thoughtful making your rank list.

## Whitney Alduron, Anesthesia

After interviews, I only ended up writing thank you notes to two of the eight programs (they both ended up being my top two), but I suppose it was more because I started to get lazy and figured it wouldn't make too much of a difference. Residents at a few of the programs actually told me not to even bother writing thank you notes because it wouldn't matter. Some programs explicitly told me that I would not hear from them before match day. They did not send out emails letting you know you had a matching spot at their program, but you could feel free to communicate your interest with them. One program actually sent me a thank you note for coming which I thought was nice.

Out of all the programs I applied to, there was only one program I was very disappointed I did not get an interview at. I spoke with my advisor and asked what I should do. He suggested I talk to another faculty member within the department and ask them to send an email on my behalf. I did, but I never heard anything after that. I am not sure whether he forgot to email them or they responded back and said no, but either way I did not get an end up getting an interview there.

> *"Call me a masochist, but I ranked the program that poisoned me first."*
>
> *-Samuel Austin*

I have to admit, it did feel awkward to ask my advisor (who is the program director here) to help me get an interview at another program because I was also very interested in staying at my home program. It just seemed as though I was giving off conflicting messages when saying "I want to stay here," but at the same time asking to get interviews at different programs. However, I have to say that my advisor did an excellent job saying that he was both my advisor and the program director, and would do whatever it takes to help me get where I want to go.

At the end of the interview season, I ended up sending one program an email saying that I planned on ranking them number one. I sent one more email to a second program saying they were at the "top of my list" because I would be ranking them number two. I did not hear back from either program after the emails. I don't know how much of a difference sending the emails made, but I told myself that it couldn't hurt.

I did receive one email from a program that stated they were very impressed with me during the interview day, and I would be ranked very highly and likely to match there. Receiving an email like that definitely made me feel excited and a little less worried about match day because even though they were not at the top of my list, I know I would be very happy at that program.

## Tyler van Backer, General Surgery

I wrote thank you notes a couple days after the interview. I hand-wrote notes for places I loved and sent emails to the rest. I had one program director send me a letter directly, and a couple programs use the ERAS system to contact me (although those weren't personalized like the letter). The usual was 'hi, thanks for coming. We all enjoyed meeting you, etc.'

I rotated at a program and interviewed with the PD and Chair who both promised me an interview and said to keep in touch. Never heard from the program again.

## Cameron Smith, Internal Medicine

To one of the programs that I really loved, I wrote a hand-written thank you card to my interviewer. With other programs, I usually emailed the interviewers and thanked them for their time. One month before rank lists were due, I emailed a few programs and let them know that they would be toward the top of my match list.

I don't think any programs lied to me or "messed with my head," but it is important to take everything that is said to you with a grain of salt. Program directors and interviewers can often give vague, positive responses.

## Mairin Jerome, PM & R

I sent all my interviewers and residents a thank you email, save for the last two interviews where I was disinterested and lazy. At the conclusion of interviews, I sent a letter of intent to my number 1 program for PM & R. For my top 5 programs, I also wrote follow up emails to the program directors to let them know

I really liked their programs and would be honored to match with them (I did not mention ranking in these).

I had two programs email me after my interview expressing interest in being part of my future training. I also received a phone call from one of those programs to see if I was still interested in the program. I assumed that this contact meant these programs had ranked me to match, but you can never really be sure. Technically by match rules, they're really not supposed to have this type of contact (or are encouraged not to). It was nice to get these communications, but also made me nervous that I hadn't heard from my top choices in the same way.

I had two different advisors call and/or write on my behalf to programs prior to interview invitations, and I was subsequently interviewed at those programs. I think it is really helpful, particularly if you had a big red flag on your application (like board failure, in my case). I also know of another applicant who called a program that apparently was waiting for applicants to express specific interest. After he called, he was invited to interview. There are 2 programs I wish in retrospect that I had called myself or asked someone to call on my behalf.

# Making The Rank List

## Alyssa Mendelson, General Surgery

I started with an excel spreadsheet that I would fill out after my interviews. Categories were "number of residents, salary, $ for food, research year(s), etc. etc." I abandoned this in about a week. There is too much information. At the end of your interview, write down one or two things you thought were unique or totally sucked about the program, and then a line or two on the gut feeling/impression of the program. I promise at the end the little details won't matter. You'll make your decision based off of your overall impression of the program.

I've gone back and forth with my #1 and #2. I haven't officially submitted a rank list yet. I'm taking as much time as I can to mull it over, and doing second looks to make sure. I haven't sent out the "You're my #1 program" letter, and I'm not sure I want to. I don't like that we are supposed to do this. Then, if a program doesn't get a letter from me, they assume they're not high on my list? I can't send another letter saying "you're high on my list!" without letting them know they aren't my #1 if I don't explicitly say "you're my #1." What a stupid concept.

Gut feeling, gut feeling, and gut feeling. After gut feeling came geography. Is this close to family and friends? Can my boyfriend visit me easily? Do I have a place to run and ski? It really depends on what's most important to you.

I didn't have anyone make any phone calls or emails on my behalf because my home program is very high on my rank list (1 or 2). That being said, I didn't want to ask them to call my other first choice/second choice program to encourage them to take me, because I didn't want to risk losing my position on my home rank list. Bummer for me.

## G. Michael Krauthamer, Emergency Medicine

When it comes time to choose a program, I heard time and again to "go with my gut." All other things being equal this seems like fair advice. In my case it was tempered by my desire to be near family, landing a job that would allow me to pay my rent and save money, and go somewhere where my partner would also be happy. So, ultimately, the decision reflects a balance of practical and gut decisions. That said, I made sure to write down a few thoughts on my gut reaction to programs immediately after an interview day. This allowed me to go back and revisit my feelings about a program, after the initial feeling faded. I tried to keep track of things like: did the residents seem happy? Tired? Cynical? Enthusiastic? Did they exhibit a sense of ownership over their program? What were the facilities like; could I see myself working there? Was the program director approachable, supportive, intimidating? These things will be hard to evaluate objectively, because programs are trying to recruit you so they'll put their best face forward. That said, the really malignant programs will not be able to hide; the day will feel disorganized, you'll feel like your interview is low priority, and the residents will seem unhappy—in short your gut will be right.

## Samuel Austin, Anesthesia

I judged places heavily on the attributes of the interviewers. Are they robotic and uninteresting? Are they interviewing candidates because they want to shape the program into the best one it can be? Once I left the interviewers were what I remembered, and, quite literally, became the faces of the program. When interviewers were selling their program too hard, it seemed desperate and was a turn-off, which is likely a reflection of my own arrogance more than anything.

One program asked me where I was interviewing later that week. It seemed benign and so wasn't off-putting. Maybe I'm a sucker.

It's funny. I was absolutely sure of my first choice after the third interview. Each program I visited after that felt almost like an afterthought. Your initial biases toward programs will likely change as you see more places; your "must have" criteria are a moving target. I struggled a lot after interviews trying to decide which of my two favorite places would get put in the top spot, and in the end, I ranked the latter program, not the one I was initially dead-set on. I realized that happiness will likely follow wherever I go, because like Kid Rock prophetically proclaimed, "you get what you put in."

Big name programs have sex appeal. But Hopkins or Penn doesn't guarantee success if you aren't willing to put in the time to become great. People at small community programs could probably out-anesthetize some of the players at the gilded institutions simply based on their work ethic. Nearly every program will give you adequate training because they're all regulated by the same governing body, so choose what you think is the best fit. Though the neurons in your enteric nervous system number a mere tenth of that in your brain, while ordering your rank list it is a good time to let the underdog do the thinking and go with your gut.

Finally, there will probably be times when you kick yourself for ranking things the way you did, but in the end it's all gravy. The grass is always greener on the other side.

Tell your #1 program they're #1. They use the metric of how far down their list they had to go as a marker of success. Everyone likes the feeling of a sure thing. I honestly have no idea whether it changes your position on their list, but I can't imagine it hurting you.

Great advice was to put all of the programs I went to into a cereal box and pull them out one-by-one and record my immediate reaction to each. This will reveal your snap judgment about the place, which can be telling.

## Burt Johnson, Urology

It's unsatisfying and seemingly unscientific, but the reality is that it's about the gut feeling. I didn't take any notes during interviews. I just evaluated programs in my head and occasionally would write two or three things down after the interview day when I got back to my hotel. Two or three positives, and two or three negatives – let me save you the drama, there is not a perfect program. My decision to go to urology in the first place was based on advice by Dr. Neil Hyman, a colorectal surgeon, and I continued to take his advice when it came down to selecting programs. His advice was to "find your people." At the end of the day a lot of it came down to my original priorities for applying to programs: geography and overall happiness. Would I be happy at a program? That was a question I was trying to answer at interviews.

Everyone is also trying to answer, "will this place trained me to be a great internists, surgeon, or whatever," but the reality is it's very difficult to know. Ask your advisor or department chair at your home program and find out from what programs they would love to hire. Find out the places they trust and believe train good people.

At the end of the day, my rank list was based on same things that were priorities at the start of the application process. I learned much about the intricacies and philosophies of programs on interview trail from other applicants. This was helpful in excluding/including programs that I previously was interested in for geographic, academic, and training reasons. I honestly felt like I would get amazing training at any of my top 7 programs. Thus, my rank list was based upon personal life situation, geography, quality of training, and quality of life. It wasn't scientific and for most people it won't be.

I didn't change my rank list at the very last second, but I was deliberating between the top two for the last week prior to certifying my rank list. Most people will tell you that you shouldn't changes at the last second, and I'd agree. Ideally, I would have certified my rank list before programs submit theirs. Technically the programs submit their rank lists at the same time as the applicants, but in talking to program directors, they usually have a meeting a month in advance and make their final rank then.

If you want to tell programs that they are your #1, you need to decide weeks before the actual official rank lists are submitted. It doesn't do you any good to tell a program two days before the deadline that they're your first choice. You might as well not tell them. There is nothing they can do about it.

## Whitney Alduron, Anesthesia

When making my rank list, all of the programs I interviewed at were very good and I knew I would get an excellent education. Simply, I had to decide where I wanted to live for the next 4 to 5 years. Some of the programs were very large (20+ residents per class) and others were very small (less than 6). Ideally I was looking for a class-size between 10 to 12, but in the end that did not end up being the biggest deciding factor.

For me it came down to geography. I have always lived in New England, and I wanted to move away for a few years and see someplace new. I have to say if you don't overthink things, the rank list is easy to make – I just put down the places I wanted to live in that order. However, as time went on and I began thinking about name recognition/reputation things got more complicated. I found myself beginning to toy with the idea of putting programs I felt were slightly out of my reach at the top of my list. Yet, I was secretly hoping I wouldn't match at those programs.

There was a little part of me that thought it was a waste of my talent/education/ hard work/etc. not to rank the most competitive program number one even if it was not my favorite. Don't play mind games like this!! It will only drive you crazy!! You need to put down programs in the order that you actually want to go to. Even though 4 years does not seem long, and you figure you can put up with anything, you are better off being at a place you will enjoy.

For most of us residency is also an important time with regards to our personal lives. This is the time when maybe you are thinking about getting married, starting a family, or even just getting a dog. In the back of your mind, you have to consider these aspects of your life when ranking programs.

## Tyler van Backer, General Surgery

Usually, I would go with a gestalt gut feeling and write it down, then used a more objective checklist from UPenn's med school that was online (http://www. med.upenn.edu/student/documents/PSOMGuidetoResidencyClassof2014.pdf). I also took faculty/alumni feedback into account, as well. Doximity just published rankings for surgery, but I'm not sure how useful they really are or on what factors they're based.

A lot came down to geography and where I felt like I would succeed in residency. I was surprised by the number of programs that disappointed me. I didn't think too much about exploring the surrounding area on interview day, so it was harder for me to know if my significant other would be happy in the locations I was ranking.

My advisor offered to send emails to people he knew at my top choice, which was awesome. My Chair offered to make calls to my top two choices. I felt semi-awkward asking, but less so since they made the first offer to do it. I think having another person vouch for you can't be anything but helpful, especially if the person went to school with/knows well/sits on a board with the PD/assistant PD/chair/etc.

I didn't change my list because I made a bunch of them prior to certifying my list. I knew that I would be tempted to change it every five minutes as fleeting thoughts came through if I didn't promise myself to keep it as it was.

## Mairin Jerome, PM & R

I started off taking notes. Then I got lazy and stopped taking notes. When making my rank list, I wished I had kept taking detailed notes. Ideally, I should have made a spreadsheet of all important components in PM & R and take 10 minutes to fill it out after each interview.

Pretty quickly during the interview day I had a sense of the program and whether or not I would fit in there. For those in the middle of my list, it would have been great to have kept better notes. I did, however, use the PRISM NRMP app on my smart phone and rated each program afterwards. I found it helpful and you can customize it to what's important to you. I shuffled it around a little afterwards, but it was helpful for keeping track of my gut reactions and not as labor intensive as opening a computer and documenting.

I knew when my #1 choice was meeting to create its rank list, and I wrote the program director (with program coordinator cc'd) a letter of intent before the meeting. I was a little nervous about this, as I had not finished all my interviews, but if the letter is going to help at all, it is best to have it in before the rank list is being made.

# 12

# POTPOURRI & STORY TIME

## Whitney Alduron, Anesthesia

Medical students love to stress about everything- starting from MCAT scores, which medical school to go to, classroom grades, board scores, residency program etc., but at the end of the day all that really matters is your happiness. It really doesn't matter where you go to medical school or where you go to residency as long as it's a place where you get a good education, enjoy work, and have a fulfilling life outside of the hospital.

As an older applicant (30 yo) I really do find myself favoring more lifestyle aspects of residency programs and the geographic location over everything else. Honestly most of the programs I interviewed at were all extremely similar: the residents were very happy (almost too happy), the work hours were the same, the schedules were very similar, the education was excellent, and board pass rates were the same. Therefore, the deciding factors were the geography and the overall feeling I got when I walked out of the hospital after my interview day.

## Burt Johnson, Urology

I failed my first exam of medical school. Don't let that stand in your way.

## Mairin Jerome, PM & R

1. I would have taken more time in preclinical years to shadow or have at least a little experience in fields with less clerkship exposure (PM & R, ophthalmology, dermatology, urology). You have time to do this in the preclinical years, and it will help you plan if you end up liking those fields. Also, a little time early on will help you forge connections with potential future advisors and/or letter writers.

2. Don't let the constant evaluation and feelings of being less than eat your soul. You are probably still a good person even if you are not at the top of your medical school class!!

3. Exercise, eat well, get enough rest, and don't lose sight of who you are. In the end, it is all worth it. Interviewing is actually really fun, though tiring. Fourth year is amazing, and it's a good time to regroup and just tidy up loose ends. Relax and have fun. Soon you will be in residency and your freedom for this will be limited.

Make time for therapy if you need it.

## Tyler van Backer, General Surgery

Good advice: relax. Interviews are stressful enough. No need to get yourself wound up thinking about the interview ahead of time. If you appear calm and relaxed, you'll also be less likely to stumble over your words and babble on forever about irrelevant minutia.

Get a good night sleep the night before. For me, that was important because there were some awful hotel beds that I couldn't sleep on and sometimes the pre-interview dinner ended up going until 10.

Ask your advisor/PD/ what the weaknesses in your application are, (we all have them) and try to have them addressed ahead of time. Highlight lessons learned and how you're preventing failures/weaknesses in the future. Remember that you're interviewing the program, too, so make sure to get the information that's important to you, as well from the day and evening prior.

## Alyssa Mendelson, General Surgery

We all will feel like a failure at some point. You tried hard to honor a class and didn't. You were supposed to call your mom for her birthday and forgot because you were studying. You'll get in fights with your significant other, your family, and your friends. Life happens in medical school. Just accept that you're doing your best and shit gets hard sometimes. Try not to beat yourself up over it.

In your clinical years, you make mistakes a lot – inside and outside the hospital. Learning early how to have some of this stuff roll off your back is important.

## Harold Callahan, Dermatology

The Callahan two pronged approach:

1. Understand the ERAS filters that residency directors use to filter applications – determining which they read and eventually which students they will interview.

2. The goal is to have as many continuous rankings (i.e. interviews that you attend) as possible. This is the single most important factor to matching in all fields. The final step is getting them to rank you highly.

## G. Michael Krauthamer, Emergency Medicine

I started medical school with the intention of applying to Psychiatry residency, and it wasn't until August of my fourth year that I decided to apply to Emergency Medicine residencies. This sort of complicated my application process because it meant identifying mentors fairly late in the process, and ultimately, it also meant figuring out how to convey to programs that I was serious about pursuing EM, despite my late arrival to the specialty.

In fact, I actually started putting together applications for both specialties, and considered applying to residencies in psychiatry and EM. However, after posting all of my materials for both specialties to ERAS, I ultimately decided to submit materials exclusively to EM programs. In part I did this to simplify my life, and because I was told by my advisors that applying to two specialties would detract from my applications, since doing so would convey a lack professional clarity (I subsequently discovered that while students from American allopathic medical schools rarely apply to two specialties, students from Caribbean schools frequently apply to two or more specialties for residency).

If you are like me and have a ninth-inning change of heart there are several things you must do: First, contact the specialty advisor at your school and find out if your chosen specialty has any special application requirements. For example, most EM programs request standardized letters of recommendation (SLOEs), ideally from EM rotations at hospitals with residency programs.

## Alyssa Mendelson, General Surgery

Females: Wear comfortable shoes! And invest in a pair that won't fall apart. My heel broke during one of mine and I couldn't walk during the tour…I hobbled back to my suitcase and had to put on my Danskos. New York City was not impressed by my fashion sense.

On that note, dress code. Please, please, please wear something simple and classic.

Suit: Navy suit. Black – you look like you're going to a funeral. Dark grey is fine, I guess. I've heard a skirt suit is better for females – old school surgeons think females should wear skirts – sexist, but I don't want that to be a reason I don't get considered for a position at a high-powered program…

Shirt: Simple, ivory, or colored shirt under your suit coat, nothing crazy or sparkly.

Jewelry: Simple earrings. Some people wore necklaces. I heard some females had a "conversational piece" that they would wear. Someone wore their Gold Human-ism pin. That seems weird to me. I had enough to talk about without a piece of jewelry speaking for me.

Make-up: Don't make your face look like you're about to walk down the runway at a fashion show. Cat-eye eyeliner? Really?

Shoes: I wore plain black, 1.5-2 inch pumps for shoes. For two interviews, I wore my kitten heel nude pumps just because they were more comfortable.

Things I saw people wear: tweed skirt, sequin silver shirt, snakeskin 4 inch heels and hoop earrings. No, no, no and no. What do you want people to remember about you? What you say or what you wore? Standing out might not be worth it in this setting.

# Story Time

## Dena Darby, Family Medicine

At one interview day, we were presented with very nice, heavy ceramic mugs with the program's name on the side. The program coordinator encouraged us to drink some coffee from them, showing us to the break room and providing cream and sugar.  Near the end of the day, I washed the mug and started gathering my papers and pens, placing the mug in my bag. As the other applicants put their coats on and gathered their belongings, I glanced at the table and noticed that all of the other applicants had left their mugs on the table. I removed my mug from my bag and placed it on the table, red-faced, glancing around to see if anyone had noticed. I'll never know if anyone did notice, but I felt uncomfortable with my misunderstanding of the situation and no one graciously said, "Please, take these mugs to remember us as you make your rank list!"

I received other free tokens throughout the season, from a small flashlight for my stethoscope to a free ice cream cone coupon, all clearly emblazoned with the program's name and symbol. I did not refuse these items and actually really enjoy using my tri-highlighter (although they are reminiscent of pharmaceutical pandering).

## Samuel Austin, Anesthesia

Best question I was asked: if there were literally no need for medicine anymore – everyone is completely healthy – what would you do? I told them I'd love to play music for a living. It was a toss-up between rock star and rally car racer, but let's be honest: rockers get all the chicks.

There are going to be ups and downs. The interview trail is at once exhilarating and exhausting. While in a city that quite literally could not have been geographically farther away from my home I came down with a wicked stomach virus – which I and twenty others had gotten – from an interview lunch the previous day. I puked almost all weekend. As shitty as getting sick was, sharing our diarrhea stories made for a great way to bond with other interviewees who had also fallen ill at the next dinner a couple days later (at which the chief resident was kind enough to order ginger ale and plain noodles for me). The program emailed all of us and apologized – maybe we got a sympathy bump on their rank list? Call me a masochist, but I ranked the program that poisoned me first.

Indeed, getting ill was a blessing in disguise, as I was able to catch up on tons of Netflix and rest. You will likely find yourself in locales that have so much to do and with precious little time to enjoy it. It can be hard to not feel pressured to do it all during your stay, but don't sacrifice too much sleep to experience the city. Getting sick allowed me to just chill and catch up. Traveling takes more energy than you might imagine. Do enjoy yourself, but make sleep a priority. Also bring some ondansetron if you can get your hands on it.

## Jennifer Tango, Emergency Medicine

### Confidence

We were supposed to meet at the University Hospital for a tour the night before the interview. I hurried into the lobby next to the piano where we were told to meet. I didn't see anyone who looked ready for a tour, but there was a group of people sitting down in plush chairs next to the piano. I rushed past them and followed the signs towards the emergency department, thinking that I may have missed the tour and if I did, perhaps I could catch up to them. I got to the entry to the ED with no sign of a tour group. I decided to go back to the piano.

The group sitting by the piano turned out to be the emergency folks interviewing the following day. Now, this was my second to last interview, and I felt quite seasoned. I had grown tired of being the first to introduce myself. Many times, I started speaking with someone who didn't explain their role, and ended up being an applicant rather than a resident.

Finally, one of the girls spoke up and said, "Hi, my name is Erin, I'm one of the applicants." "Hi!" I said. "I'm Jen. I'm also applying." Everyone looked super surprised and then all seemed to relax a bit. It turns out that they all thought I was one of the residents and that I was going to be the one leading the tour! "You walked up here looking like you knew what was up and were ready to take charge!"

An important lesson, not just for interviewing for residency, but for life in general is that you will go a lot further if you have confidence.. You have to know that the program is not just interviewing you, but more importantly, you are interviewing them. Having this perspective takes the pressure off the interview.

A program director made a comment to me that there are no bad emergency medicine residency programs in the US, there are only bad fits. I think this is so true, and probably generally true for all residency types.

### My First Interview

I was extremely nervous for my first interview and didn't really want to show up alone. I thought it would be better to carpool with someone, and have a companion before getting thrown into the lion's den. One of the other applicants offered a ride, and we planned to meet in the lobby of my hotel. After sitting there for over 50 minutes, she finally texted me saying that she was 20 minutes away. "What the crap?"

When she finally arrived 30 minutes later, I got in her car filled with clutter, junk, and pungent odor. Still, I thought to myself that I was glad I was not driving. She pulled out into traffic, a car swerved to avoid us, and she proceeded to cut a corner too sharp and hit the curb…ker-thunk…

Though it probably wasn't then, I think my favorite part of this story now was the windshield wipers. This girl had her windshield wipers on full blast, as if we were in a hurricane, and it wasn't even raining.

I tell this story for a couple reasons. First, you don't know these people! Be careful whose vehicle you enter. I can't imagine a worse introduction to the emergency department at your future residency program than getting in a wreck, getting brought to the hospital by EMS and having someone staring at you from above, saying "Hello! Welcome to our Emergency Department! We are with the trauma team and are going to cut your clothes off you now!"

Second, I think it is very telling about a program when the program director takes time to know your application and memorizes your name and picture so that they can recognize you. I knew this was the kind of program for me, where people actually care if you become a good doctor or not.

## Mairin Jerome, PM & R

Punctuality is not my forte. I tended to not leave enough time to get to my interviews. I was 15 minutes late for an interview in Atlanta, missed the talk from the chair of the department, and walked in during the middle of the presentation from the program director. This was a program I was really interested in. That is poor form. I had no idea there would be a ton of traffic in Atlanta at 6:30am. So, give yourself a lot of extra time and plan ahead. I don't think it counts majorly against you (I saw people come in late a few times and it wasn't a huge deal), but definitely better to be early. At one interview, one guy showed up 30 minutes late and program director was really nice and waited until he arrived to start the day. So we were all waiting around for this guy for 30 minutes. When he finally strolled in, he made an offhanded comment, and didn't even apologize for being late. If you are late, apologize.

I am an older applicant (age 32 at time of interviewing), and when it comes time to interview, this was an asset. I have a unique perspective and generally a broader range of experiences than younger applicants. One is not better than the other, but it made interviewing pretty easy because I had a lot of experiences to draw on. If you are an older applicant, make sure you provide a clear verbal outline of your path. Because of the way applications are printed, it is difficult for interviewers to follow the timeline.

## Burt Johnson, Urology

Before you go to your interviews be sure to double check where to show up. I had previously been to Hartford Hospital and knew it was the main teaching hospital for UConn's program. Foolishly, I assumed that the interview day would be held there. I arrived at the hospital about 15 minutes before start time and asked the information desk where the urology interviews were being held. I was directed to a bunch of applicants sitting at a table across the atrium. I walked over and asked the applicants if they were here for the urology interviews and they said, "Yup, we're here for the neurology interviews!"

At that point I went back to information and asked for the residency coordinator and made sure to place a phone call saying that I would be late and that I was at the wrong place. I arrived about half an hour into the department chair's presentation, quite embarrassing.

## Calvin Barber, Anesthesia

I'm loving fourth year, and it's because I am really making an effort to do stuff that is interesting to me with absolutely no thought of whether it makes my application look stronger or weaker or anything else. So I'm currently doing virtual reality medicine which is just… so out there. I got involved with that just because of somebody I got talking to at a conference and it seemed really interesting, cutting edge, and might be fun to spend a month doing.

I also did a mission surgical mission to Guatemala which was incredible. Fourth year is the chance to play, and I really recommend taking that chance.

# NOTES

# NOTES

# INDEX

## A

Whitney Alduron  3, 15, 18, 27, 31, 38, 43, 45, 50, 53, 57, 71, 83, 88, 94, 101, 102, 112, 119, 125, 130, 133

Samuel Austin  3, 13, 23, 25, 42, 43, 44, 53, 57, 61, 66, 72, 80, 91, 93, 98, 100, 103, 111, 114, 118, 122, 125, 128, 137

## B

Calvin Barber  3, 15, 17, 19, 30, 31, 35, 40, 48, 51, 55, 69, 75, 77, 78, 91, 94, 103, 105, 140

## C

Harold Callahan  3, 12, 18, 20, 27, 32, 38, 56, 60, 66, 70, 74, 82, 92, 94, 99, 135

## D

Dena Darby  3, 12, 110, 112, 115, 117, 124, 137

## J

Mairin Jerome  3, 14, 22, 29, 33, 37, 46, 49, 53, 54, 64, 73, 87, 88, 89, 96, 99, 103, 110, 115, 120, 126, 132, 134, 139

Burt Johnson  3, 10, 13, 18, 26, 32, 36, 41, 47, 61, 68, 76, 79, 89, 94, 105, 113, 118, 123, 129, 134, 140

## K

G. Michael Krauthamer  3, 13, 39, 52, 63, 67, 74, 75, 79, 93, 108, 114, 122, 128, 135

## M

Alyssa Mendelson  3, 14, 16, 24, 25, 36, 44, 48, 49, 53, 54, 60, 65, 68, 74, 81, 90, 92, 99, 100, 102, 104, 108, 113, 117, 120, 121, 127, 135, 136

## N

Hank Ng  3, 12, 22, 27, 32, 34, 51

## S

Cameron Smith  3, 14, 20, 29, 33, 36, 44, 50, 59, 72, 73, 86, 91, 96, 102, 103, 116, 120, 126

## T

Jennifer Tango  3, 15, 21, 63, 96, 138

## V

Tyler van Backer  3, 15, 21, 28, 33, 37, 46, 50, 52, 58, 71, 73, 84, 90, 97, 99, 100, 102, 110, 116, 119, 121, 126, 131, 134

# THANK YOU

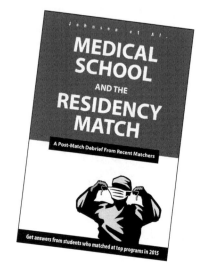

Thank you very much for reading this book, we all sincerely hope you have taken something of value from it. Our goal was simply to fill a need for present and future medical students. Therefore, if you feel that some of the information is outdated, inaccurate, or complete hogwash, please let us know.

Additionally, if you feel that you have some unique perspectives to contribute, please get in touch as well as the book is updated annually to reflect the most accurate and recent information. There are opportunities for prospective authors to contribute in fields that have less information in this book.

## Your Feedback

Please let us know what your thoughts were on the book. If you felt it was worthy of a 5-star review on Amazon, please support us with that! If you thought it needed work in some areas, please contact us through the contact page at www.MedicalMatchBook.com so that we can put out a new and improved edition.

Thank you so much for supporting this student-created product!

| | |
|---|---|
| Web Site | www.MedicalMatchBook.com |
| Facebook | www.facebook.com/medicalmatch |
| Amazon | amzn.com/1514205386 |

Made in the USA
Middletown, DE
30 June 2015